Making it to Kindergarten

Making it to Kindergarten

A Race to Save Landon from Autism

Laurie Hilton

NSP

NORTH STONINGTON
PRESS

MAKING IT TO KINDERGARTEN

North Stonington Press

Copyright © 2018
Laurie Hilton

Ordering Information: bookpatch.com
Website: makingittokindergarten.com

For permission request, visit: makingittokindergarten.com

First Edition

ISBN: 978-1-7321412-0-9 (Paperback)
ISBN: 978-1-7321412-1-6 (eBook)

Library of Congress information available
LCCN: 2018907057

Printed in the United States of America
10 9 8 7 6 5 4 3 2 1

Disclaimer: *The advice and treatment plans found in this
book may not be suitable for every situation. This book is sold with
the understanding that neither the author nor publisher are held responsible for
any actions taken that may result in damage or loss. This book is not intended
as a substitute for the medical advice of physicians. The reader should regularly
consult a physician in matters relating to his/her health or child's health
and particularly with respect to any symptoms that may
require diagnosis or medical attention.*

Dedicated to Landon: You fought and won the hardest battle of your life. You are my champion and my inspiration.

CONTENTS

Foreword i

Introduction iii

1   Seeing the Signs 1

2   Leaky Gut 13

3   Oh My Candida 33

4   Biomedical Treatment Begins 45

5   Man on Fire Syndrome/Coconut Kefir 51

6   Diet 71

7   B12 Injections 79

8   Regression 87

9   Holistic Try 99

10   It's in the Stars 105

11   Superhero 109

12   Blood Draw 117

13   I Know 133

14   Light at the End of the Tunnel 139

15   The Final Breakthrough 149

16   Tummy Still Hurts 161

17   Back to Connecticut 165

18   You Scoop the Poop, I Make the Soup, ... 173

19   Go Carts, Bicycles, and Bumper Cars 179

20   The Finish Line 183

21   To Ed 195

Epilogue 197

Credits 201

References 203

About the Author 206

FOREWORD

Our digestive system is home to the body's defensive (immune) system. It is the key to our health. When the digestive system breaks down, your immune system begins to show signs of failure, affecting every function of your body from your brain and liver, to your thyroid, to your blood and metabolism. Most people do not know that all diseases or disorders can be traced back to an unhealthy gut, such as in this case, autism. However, did you know whatever health issue you have (whether it be Alzheimer's dementia, schizophrenia, or even cancer) can be turned around and reversed by first focusing on repair of the digestive system? This is the basic precept of my podcast "The Bright Side with Ben Fuchs," a syndicated radio program on the GCN Radio Network.

The author of this book and mother of Landon, Laurie Hilton, is an avid listener of my show, and I am pleased that it was through listening to my show that she was able to learn and apply some basic treatments of dealing with the gut-brain connection, and later see real improvements in her son Landon's condition.

Years back, when Laurie called my show, she disclosed personal details about Landon's health; primarily eczema, allergies, and intestinal pain at the time. She was unaware many of the symptoms she was seeing was actually a breakdown of her son's immune system, degenerating into autism. Many of the doctors she took him to only provided her with temporary symptom relief solutions which didn't target the cause of his condition, Leaky Gut.

So I gave her advice on the air about some supplements and foods she could use to help her son's Leaky Gut. She has been able to use many of my suggestions, and has promised to keep in touch with me periodically to stay updated on his progress. After many trials and tribulations, and persistence through adversity, Landon was finally able to show improvement in his condition, and miraculously almost all of his autistic symptoms he was showing have disappeared. Landon's recovery is a great example of how through nutrition and supplementation your body can overcome many diseases. This story is not only about autism, it is about digestive health and health in general. I hope that his example shines through to anyone else who may face similar bodily issues, and act as a road map for healing.

You might find personal connections you can relate to in this book. By applying common sense and a solid nutritional plan, you too may see improvements in your own health, and also the health of your loved ones.

Ben Fuchs

Host of "*The Bright Side*" with Ben Fuchs
Founder of Truth Treatments Skin Care products

INTRODUCTION

Make it to kindergarten, a feat so absurdly easy it can hardly be considered a goal. Or is it that easy? Ask any parent of an autistic child and it can sound like climbing Mt. Everest. This simple goal started as a journey for us, and this journey became a race, a desperate race to save our son's life. You will see this story is about a boy pushed to his limits, and his taxing struggle to overcome his health challenges.

In this book I will talk about the steps we took to save our son's ailing health and reverse his neurological impairment; what is more commonly known today as autism. In essence, it became more of a dual race. Keep in mind, what worked for us may not necessarily work for your child. Each child is different and requires an individual diagnosis as well as their own protocol for healing. Landon's father and I are not doctors, and this book should not be taken as a prescription for any of you to cure any of your child's ailments. If you have a child with similar problems to ours, I encourage you to educate yourself on all of the possible causes and symptoms and talk to as many doctors as possible. It's always best to act according to your own best interests, taking into account all of your child's specific medical conditions. I wish you the same outcomes that we have had!

After months of speaking with doctors, reading and researching in books and online, we decided there was only one option for us: biomedical intervention. Since writing this book, I have noticed the labels of the doctors in this field fluctuate even though they apply the same or similar practice. Over time I have seen it change from biomedical, to integrative medicine, to MAPS, to functional medicine. I will refer to our treatment as biomedical. We chose the biomedical approach after the line of modern day medical doctors failed us. What began in a life-altering BabyCenter forum read took us through three states in our search to find the best biomedical doctors in the field. I am going to take you on our voyage so you can learn from what we experienced, and the trials and tribulations we dealt with along our passage. I will outline each step of the way; what we tried, what failed, and what succeeded. Also, I explain the significance of the changes we saw along the way on our child's path of healing. Sometimes what seemed like distressing moments actually made way for positive change. As the saying goes, often we took two steps forward, then one step back. This catchphrase could not hold more truth during our journey to heal our son Landon. Eventually the frog climbs out of the well and just like that frog, your child can do it too, but you must persevere.

You may spend many months and even years of running into roadblocks and retracing your steps when something fails to work. I remember feeling so alone and scared after leaving each doctor appointment because the truth of the matter was, we had to move mountains. Basically we had to be our own doctor, as we would learn from a radio show host. The doctor is not going to live in your house with you and hold your hand each step of the way, tracking what works or doesn't work. You have to do the hard work, but in the end the payoff may be huge. I want this book to be encouragement for you to keep following your own feelings and intuitions, and keep believing, no matter what road-blocks you come across.

I will always remember our doctor's statement to me, one so profound it became an incentive for the title of this book. "You're worried about the rest of his life...I just want to get him to kindergarten, woman!" Sometimes you need to focus on the nearest battles to win the war. If we can make it to kindergarten, we can get him anywhere. The question is, will kindergarten get there first or will we win this race?

1

SEEING THE SIGNS

'When you say unpopular things, you have got to know
who you are and believe in what you are doing."
Dr. Phil McGraw

Landon was born in Connecticut in February of 2012, and he appeared to be a healthy, beautiful child. I was divorced, with a 10 year old daughter named Angela, and my boyfriend Ed had recently moved in with us. Landon was our first child together. We were both excited to raise our baby together. Little did we know about the voyage this little boy was about to take us on, and how I may have inadvertently caused my little angel so much suffering and anguish.

I always considered myself healthy due to the fact I feverishly exercised on a daily basis and never did drugs. Occasionally I drink and yes I have my sweet tooth, however, I never could have imagined the galaxy of misinformation presented to me and the blinders I had on. In my opinion, the information I had learned along the way did not appear to exist in the mainstream medical system. It was going to be up to me to search for the answers, something that was not going to just fall into my lap. Notwithstanding everything I thought I knew, I was about to get a crash course in biology and nutrition.

The day Landon was born he was perfect. The tests leading up to his birth indicated there was a one in three chance he would have Down Syndrome. I was concerned but prepared to accept and love this baby no matter what but at the same time hoping to beat the odds. His face was flawless and with a full head of hair. When we took him home we would gaze at him all day. He slept in his swing quite a bit, appearing so serene and content. Several weeks like this passed by as I recall thinking how easy this baby was compared to Angela, my first. Little did we know the lords of bedlam were about to come calling, for our perfect little world was actually teetering on the edge of a catastrophic drop. Whether we liked it or not, our lives as we knew it were going to be shaken, bent, and turned upside down.

FIRST SIGNS

One thing I have noticed in life is that it comes at you in the most unexpected ways. Nothing happens the way you intend; instead it plays out with unpredictable twists and turns. I never thought having a child with autism was going to be part of my plan in life, and I certainly never expected this reality to manifest in the manner it did. As I walked out of the supermarket finishing my errands one morning, my phone rang, it was Ed. Usually Ed texts me unless it's more of an important matter, which I hoped was not the case today. As I put the phone up to my ear, I stopped dead in my tracks. In the background I heard mayhem, more like bone chilling screeches. It was a cry unlike any cries I had ever heard a baby make before, as if it were life and death. Ed could not tell me what was wrong as I ran to my car to race home. While still on the phone with Ed I was trying to get answers as to what was wrong with Landon. He frantically replied, "The oven was on and started burning something. Landon just went crazy." I pleaded with Ed to take him outside immediately, away from the burning smell or smoke. He rushed outside into the fresh air and, as if on cue, Landon's cries abruptly stopped. It was a reaction so severe; it must have overloaded his senses. When I arrived home, we waited for the smell to clear out and looked inside the oven. Drippings from a sweet potato had burned the bottom and once reheated, had created the smoky smell. How odd that a burning smell could trigger such an over-the-top reaction! This same incident happened again the following day, and was met with the same hypersensitive reaction from Landon. Even though we kept the oven spotless from this point forward, making improvements in cleaning was not going to resolve what the base of Landon's problem was. We discovered his sensitivity to smell applied to most any scent above his threshold. Perfumes and even flatulence from an unknowing guest would send Landon into a squall for an hour. Additionally, we came to find out Landon was hypersensitive to sounds as well. People who would coo at him from an arm's length away would wake him and set him off into cries of terror, as if they were blowing a trumpet in his ear. Not too long after, Landon's problems were rapidly advancing to another level.

SKIN ISSUES

Although Landon started off a very content baby, the 3 month mark is where things really started to fall apart. One morning Landon woke up with what looked like a rash on his cheek. We gave it a few days but it only seemed to get worse. The rash then spread to the other cheek as well, and then started to weep liquid. We booked an appointment with the pediatrician, a 40-minute drive to East Hampton. You may ask why we had a pediatrician so far away. The truth is, we were kicked out of our local pediatrician's practice because of our refusal to vaccinate. Aside from the Vitamin K shot, Landon never received any vaccines. I had heard great reviews from a friend of mine about their pediatrician who accepted non-vaccinated children, so as a result, every appointment for us would be a rather long car trip. Before I go any further, let me state this is not an anti-vaccination book. At the time, not vaccinating Landon was the decision we made for our own private reasons.

The pediatrician prescribed a steroid cream (Hydrocortisone Valerate Cream USP), which we applied for the next several days. The cream helped a little bit at first, but the rash came back with a fury several weeks later. The eczema had now spread from his ankles and calves all the way up to his wrists. I had eczema as a child so I could not help but think it was a genetic condition that Landon inherited from me. We assumed at this point this was something more than eczema; it looked more like a staph infection. After several more trips back to the doctor nothing in his condition had changed, even with adding an antibiotic for the infection and using a stronger topical steroid. His poor cheeks had to be constantly patted down and he was scratching all over like a fiend. Why was this eczema so out of control? It became so bad, when Landon went to bed at night we put socks over his hands and hair bands around his ankles so he could not scratch. The alternative was ripped open skin, bloody sheets, and more infections. The eczema became the main focus of our attention. Why was he so infested with these skin lesions and wildfire eczema?

All I knew at this point was what I had been told, never bothering to look elsewhere for alternative possible answers for myself. Is it possible that eczema is a manifestation of what is going on inside your body and little to do with the skin itself? I believe now that is a very plausible opinion to consider, but I did not at the time. Throughout my life I was told eczema is genetic, and will pass as we age. Landon's eczema hardly seemed genetic, and only appeared to be alleviated with creams and ointments temporarily. Little did we know, several life-changing steps had to be taken for this to resolve (stay tuned). We must have kept CVS and Walgreens in business for a good year buying up their entire department of topical ointments, attempting to rid Landon of this skin problem once and for all, but nothing worked.

ALLERGIES & FOOD INTOLERANCES

Another dangerous issue that presented itself was that Landon became allergic and intolerant to everything but air: dairy, peanuts (anaphylactic), beef, chicken, carrots, peas, everything jarred or packaged...you name it. Everything he ate gave him either a rash or intestinal discomfort, episodes I will discuss in detail later on. The only foods he could eat were bananas, squash, raisins and eggplant. His intestinal tract was obviously a mess.

Around the 6 month-old stage, Landon began crying louder than usual. Holding him did not seem to help. The crying continued as we took him downstairs and walked around passing it off as colic. The days only got worse from here as the colic transitioned to back arching while screaming. It was obviously a sign of pain, but where was it coming from? I went over in my head what we fed him that day and through process of elimination the only thing different I came up with was jarred baby food pears. I decided I would not buy pears anymore or that brand of baby food.

As the weeks wore on, those cries became high intensity screams and this is where true life-threatening fear started to set in. We knew at this point normal pampering and care was not good enough and this loss of control put us in unknown territory. On top of the eczema issue, I was scheduling one appointment after another for this intestinal issue as well. Out of their league of training, the pediatrician ultimately referred Landon to a dermatologist for his skin condition. When it came to the intestinal problem, the pediatricians served little to no effect at all. I vaguely recall acid reflux as their answer to the cause of his internal pain, which we treated with children's antacid with little to no success. The intestinal issue became worse over the course of the following weeks as the cries of agony became exorcist-like, and more frequent. The high-pitched screaming was accompanied with back arching, body jerking, writhing and flailing. The fear we had from several weeks ago now turned to sheer panic.

As the dermatologist appointment approached, I talked to Ed about my fears of going. Landon's screaming and crying seemed to incorporate most of the day and I did not think we could make the drive, let alone get through the appointment. I sat and stared for several minutes at the car seat as I contemplated canceling the appointment. We had gone so far as to tailor the car seat to Landon's skin condition. The neck rest along with the entire car seat was covered with hypo-allergenic cloth that Ed had fastened with safety pins. I could not help but think everything we were doing was reacting. We were metaphorically and literally applying band-aids.

How was this addressing the fundamental cause of this problem?

I knew deep down inside the appointment would be a waste of time, another band-aid to a plaguing, out-of-reach problem. Regardless of my feelings, I made the drive. The dermatologist introduced herself and explained apologetically that she was hard of hearing, so bear with her. This proved to be a blessing in disguise, for Landon spared no victims that day. As he screamed his lungs out like a child possessed, it became an almost impossible feat to last even five minutes of that appointment. I remember the unforgettable look of horror on that doctor's face as I ran out the door. Miraculously, before I left, she was able to prescribe some stronger medical topical steroids, specifically Fluticasone Propionate Ointment .005% and Desonide Ointment .05%.

She also wrote a prescription out for Nutramigen, a baby formula that was dairy free. I did not argue with the doctor. I thought maybe I would intermittently breastfeed while giving him this formula supplementally. Since he seemed allergic to my milk, I had to pretty much eliminate every food known to mankind in order to feed him. This would turn out to be one of the biggest regrets I've ever had. Not a day goes by I don't feel some type of guilt for taking him off my milk and onto formula.

We kept Landon on formula for about the next eight months because that was virtually all he could eat, and it supplied him with nutrients. To summarize, he was breast fed from birth to six months with sporadic formula feeds and then switched to formula for the next eight months.

Aside from the daily screams and chaos that had taken over our lives, he seemed to be developing normally in terms of walking and doing other baby milestones, but then things just spiraled downward. Well past his first year, we noticed Landon walking off balance and crashing into objects right in front of him. He would topple over a lot as if drunk, and run into things that seemed easily avoidable. Ed would pass it off as a normal for his age because he was approaching the toddler stage and that is what they do...toddle. This just did not seem normal to me, because it seemed as well, that Landon was choosing to cry over talking at all.

I'm not sure why it never occurred to me as odd (after having already raised my first child), but Landon never did babble or point. I thought he said "Angela" once at three months, or something resembling my daughter's name. Fears about autism set in and I consumed myself with the internet with each passing day. I researched every problem he had and each time I came upon a symptom, I created a reason why Landon did not have autism. He did not match all the criteria, meaning he did not have all the symptoms on these lists, only a few. We wanted to look the other way, and tell ourselves he will outgrow this. Mostly we were concerned about the pain he seemed to be in, but also he was not neurologically developing on time. Over weeks and months, I constantly immersed myself in articles about what milestones your child reach, and I knew he was not where he was supposed to be.

Waking to screams every night was now the norm and no longer the exception, but one particular night it was bad enough to wake my daughter. I can recall this as Landon's most inconsolable night yet. Normally, even the sound of a train coming through the house would not wake this girl. I remember her standing with us at 4am asking "What's wrong with him?", as we helplessly watched him roll around on the floor. After 30-40 minutes, the episode stopped and he went back to sleep. We were left with no answers; only theory and conjecture. I guess you accept any answer given to you, if only to pacify yourself for the time being, while hoping the issue passes. Well, it didn't pass, and to add to our already growing list of problems, I noticed his weight was rapidly dropping off as well.

Here we had a child suffering from skin pain and itching, while at the same time not being able to eat anything due to having either an immediate allergic reaction or a painful GI food intolerance reaction. Now in addition to the constant itching and pain, we had to worry about the weight loss and hope to figure out this mystery before it's too late. I was consumed with anxiety as I fought to organize my thoughts. Do all these issues tie into his weight loss, and what do we focus on first? I spent the next several weeks at the pediatrician's office begging for answers as to what was plaguing my child. What was causing this eczema? Why is he in so much pain? Why is he screaming like he is possessed? I needed answers now. Again, all the doctors would tell me was it could be anything from gastrointestinal distress to acid reflux, but here, have some more steroids to help with the eczema matter. Hydrocortisone was not the answer for us, not anymore. Ed once said something to me along the lines of, "Never put anything on your skin you are not willing to ingest." Maybe not being a doctor is the key to knowing something so self-evident?

We've never been a fan of pharmaceutical drugs to begin with, but something about this medication in particular scared us. The steroid cream to us was a fast answer to a larger problem. Yes, it clears the skin up in a day or two but the flare-ups appeared to get worse down the road. The last thing we wanted to do was throw gasoline on a fire. The doctors were not getting to the root of the cause. Why could they not figure out what was ailing my child? These were not normal every day issues a parent brings their child in for time and time again. This was not an average case of eczema, it was staph like. As for the intestinal issue (tell me if I am wrong) children do not normally shriek in terror and pain for hours at a time. I'm sorry but "Little Remedies" oral drops will not resolve an agonizing intestinal issue that has obviously proved itself to be more than just discomfort. The doctors were unequivocally perplexed, and it was easy for them to brush us off...this only infuriated me. There had to be an answer! I'm quite certain we were not the only ones going through this, although at times it sure did seem that way.

It's a very lonely and hopeless road to go down when you have a sick child. Nobody can help you and the answers seem out of reach. Additionally, the nighttime episodes graduated into daytime ones as well, so we had to eliminate the night terror theory. We were completely and totally bewildered. We had a sick child, we did not know what was wrong, and all we could do was stand there and watch as he physically and neurologically deteriorated away in front of us. No pediatrician could tell us what was wrong, and we did not feel as if any of them really cared. I was furious with the medical profession, as they held no credibility with me anymore. At this point, the only thing I believed they were good for were boo-boos, sniffles, and perhaps some slightly better than over-the-counter prescription strength cough medicine.

Landon was 14 months of age when it finally came...our breaking point. Everyone has a moment in their life that stays with them forever. Even years later, it's a moment you relive over and over again in your head as if it just happened. I've never had a mental or nervous breakdown, but I'm fairly certain this either was one or a close relative of one. Landon had been up all week several times during each night screaming and urinating through diapers. He was a child way beyond the brink of sanity. By the way, at this time I was pregnant with my third child, and about to give birth. I'm surprised I did not go into early labor during these weeks, with all the stress and anxiety we had been going through on a daily basis.

The screaming started again for a second time that night, startling us awake. We threw off the covers and ran into Landon's room again wondering what could be next, what dreadful thing is going to happen now? The sounds of his cries cannot be explained in words. Each minute he screamed was unbearable. It filled our hearts with agony to stand helpless and with nobody there to help us. The screams were not even screams anymore; they were blood-curdling noises that sounded as if he was being killed. I wanted to die. I wanted to take his place so he didn't have to suffer.

After 45 minutes or so of him crying, I contemplated taking him to the ER. Did we really want to subject him to an unwelcome, unhygienic hospital environment? Would they understand our situation or be just like all the rest of the doctors who shrug their shoulders, and put a temporary band-aid on? We put Landon in the car only to have him fall asleep two minutes down the road. We turned the car around and came back home. Hours later the horror started over again, and our emotions now were in maximum overdrive. As Ed tried to hold Landon, who was now thrashing around, I left his room and went downstairs pacing back and forth.

This moment was the first time in my adult life I can say I had ever experienced true powerlessness. Overcome by grief and panic, the room spun as I struggled to hold it together. Temporarily out of my mind, I left the room and remember collapsing at the bottom of the stairs while Ed held Landon. I sat bawling and heaving until Ed finally came downstairs. Landon's episode had run its course and he fell back asleep. "He went through two diapers in a matter of minutes", Ed blurted.

We sat and cried together for what seemed like hours, both of us at a loss as to how to help our son. Then another scary notion crossed my mind. I know a common symptom of diabetes is urinating profusely. Lately, during these rages, he would urinate what seemed like buckets at a time. He would also look as if he was going to pass out in his high chair at mealtimes. Both pointed to blood sugar issues, irregardless of whether or not it might be diabetes. In my mind, the future doctor visits I knew I had to make were now looking insurmountable, and more complicated to explain, as Landon's growing list of health issues began multiplying. He would surely soon be put into a failure to thrive category, and now we also had to consider the possibility he was diabetic. This became yet another ingredient to add to the combination. The following day, we would test his blood sugar.

That night, we stayed up until sunset and talked. We came to the conclusion that all the people and doctors who could not help or listen to us, would simply just blame us in the end if Landon did not improve. We had to do something, ourselves...now...or we will lose our son.

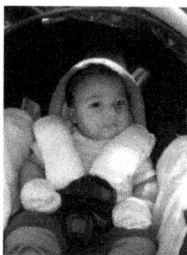

Landon with his protective coverings.

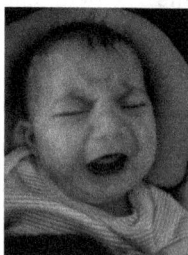

Landon with facial eczema.

2

LEAKY GUT

With Landon's health (age 14 months) and our lives in rapid descent, we happened to come upon a radio host whose words spun us in a new direction. His name was Ben Fuchs, a former pharmacist now nutritionist alerting people about the dangers of what he calls "today's medical model". He hosted a nationally syndicated daily radio show on GCN called "The Bright Side", and would prove to impact our lives in what would be a monumental way (I will be referencing Ben throughout this book). I first heard him on a radio talk show where after 15 minutes of listening, he had completely won me over. I became intrigued enough to later download his solo radio show he hosted and listen to him independently. He spoke eloquently, straightforward, and with the utmost knowledgeability. Listening to his podcast "The Bright

Side with Ben Fuchs" became a daily routine. Every day he had callers with similar problems I could relate to, so I began taking notes. We listened to his shows with an eager ear to what seemed a priceless goldmine of information. As he spoke, the wheels started spinning, and things began to click and make sense. Thus began our journey towards figuring out what was wrong with Landon.

Before each show, Ben's introduction is all about the body's natural ability to heal and repair itself as long as you give it the tools it needs. Speaking light years beyond any medical professional I have ever heard, Ben educates people about nutrition, health, biology, and supplementation. Most of the time he reveals things we had never heard before, yet the answers were right in front of us the whole time. We just needed to be awoken to them. He spoke about all diseases and ailments, and how everything wrong with us can be traced back to an unhealthy digestive system. Once your digestive system is healed and functioning properly, your body takes over and can do its job again. His upbeat dialogue always gave the listener reassurance that any disease or condition is reversible. I listened intently to his show hoping our situation would pop up, and sure enough it did not take long for eczema and allergies to be mentioned. This marked the first time I was given logical explanations and helpful suggestions. Every topic he covered began and ended with digestive health; something often overlooked and directly tied to the immune system. He describes a term called "leaky gut," which means if your digestive tract is unhealthy or damaged, certain foods you eat will cause toxins to leak out of the gut through holes into your bloodstream causing an auto immune response. I had never heard this term before and spent many days reading up on it. After reading and listening to several of his shows, it did not take long for me to realize I had destroyed Landon's gut; I had destroyed his immune system.

Ben emphasizes most mainstream doctors do not learn about the gut. They are not biochemists, therefore they are not taught how to heal. Part of his explanation for this is that doctors study clinical chemistry (involving tests), not organic chemistry within the body. So what does this mean if you have an ailment? Ben says you need to go see a biochemist if you want help with a health issue, not a doctor (In my opinion Ben ranks in the top 1% of this field worldwide). Interestingly enough, Webmd.com quotes a medical doctor in an article called "Leaky Gut Syndrome: What is it?". Gastroenterologist Donald Kirby, MD, director of the center of for Human Nutrition at the Cleveland Clinic, states: "Leaky gut syndrome isn't a diagnosis taught in medical school."[1] This did not come as a shock to me considering none of Landon's doctors up to this point had addressed the digestive system at all. Kirby also states "physicians don't know enough about the gut, which is our biggest immune system organ."[2] Forgive me for sounding logical and shrewd, but wouldn't it make sense that the curriculum in medical schools be revised to maybe center more around the digestive system? You just read a full admission from a doctor that not only is the gut our biggest immune system organ, but nothing about Leaky Gut diagnosis is taught in medical school. If the gut is our most important part of our immune system, common sense tells me here that maybe the dynamics involving the gut need to be a top priority!

Ben has an appropriate analogy comparing your health to getting your car fixed. Would you keep bringing your car back to a mechanic who never fixed your car but kept telling you to come back to patch the same problem? He asks something along the lines of, "Would you keep going back to a doctor month after month when he never does anything to heal you?" He explains, prescribed drugs only interfere with your system, they do not fix anything. An argument Ben frequently raises about prescription medications is that they stifle or shut down the body's immune response when this is your body's way of warning you of the danger you are in. In my opinion, this is so far removed from what healing is all about. Not being taught how to heal is probably why I've never seen a general practitioner ditching the prescription medications for supplements. Hence, "The Bright Side" was born. Ben says doctors do not even know what kind of dangerous substances are in the pharmaceutical drugs they prescribe. A pharmacist however, knows the ins and outs of biology/science within the body and chemistry of the drugs that are manufactured. You will find that even supplemental products we use are made by biochemists, not doctors. For instance, Ben founded Truth Treatments Systems, a line of skin supplementation products he developed himself, designed to work at the cellular level. He hints that he does not use "rare melons from South France" as the secret ingredient behind his supplemental products! My understanding of that is, there are no secrets up his sleeve as to why his products work. He is being straightforward. Since we are biochemical beings, he simply formulates his products with nutrients our bodies utilize.

WHERE YOU SEE THE PROBLEM IS NOT WHERE THE PROBLEM IS

So many things started to make sense, including my frustrations about the incompetence of the doctors we experienced. Finally I could see a shimmer of what we had going on. Revert back to Landon's pediatricians and that dermatologist who gave him a multitude of topical steroids. Nobody understood the long term effects, or considered the possibility that the problem may lie from within. Did they all go to the same substandard medical school? I doubt it. Medical schools are not teaching about the gut! I completely agree with Ben when it comes to Dermatologists even being relevant in the medical field. If the problem does lie from within, and it sure looks that way to me, this presents a problem for dermatologists and their significance in the medical community. (I'm going to go ahead and toss those pediatricians into the irrelevant pool as well, since they have proved to be nothing more than a hindrance.) Steroids, I remember Ben saying, only suppresses the immune system, something any doctor should know. Not only did this dermatologist prescribe steroids, she also prescribed a formula made for a sugar addict. This was something I subsequently learned compounded Landon's Leaky Gut issues. This whole dermatologist fiasco proved to support Ben's number one healing principle of "where you see the problem is not where the problem is".

His overall philosophy is one that puts the responsibility for your health on you, the listener. Every problem can be reversed. What I found fascinating about his show is that he had an explanation behind every condition and symptom; it was purely cause and effect. Chronically elevated cortisol and inflammation is linked to all progressive degenerative disease, therefore work on figuring out why this exists and take steps to reduce it. He spoke about fasting, eliminating all foods, then reintroducing them back one by one to see exactly which offending agent is causing a reaction, such as in cases of IBS or arthritis. Once you do this, you can target the foods that cause problems. One mission I aspired to do was three-day fasts that Ben talks regularly about. Fasting, he says, is a great way to eliminate toxins as your body starts its repair. When you eat, your body is focused on digesting and not on repairing. This is why you feel a lot better when you do not eat, noticeable even after only several hours. Landon was still too young to fast but I definitely planned on doing this for myself.

Other things about the show you may not be accustomed to hearing is that cholesterol is a fantastic thing, and so are mineral salts. He states cholesterol is the body's major building substance therefore foolish for a doctor to prescribe a drug to lower it. My doctors' thought processes have proven to be completely inverse to this, a legitimate reason why I think this show is vital for clearing up myths and disinformation. All along I have been told to watch my cholesterol when in fact I learned that foods rich in healthy fats such as butter and eggs are very good for you and not something you should want to restrict. Since learning and reading up on this, I have tripled my intake of foods with healthy fats and replaced table salt with mineral salt, an essential ingredient I learned was necessary for healthy adrenal function. With every meal now, I add Himalayan or Celtic sea salt, eat more eggs, and never deprive myself of adequate amounts of butter! Further on, I go into more detail about mineral salts. Please note, I am not telling you to do what I do. Conduct your own research to reach a conclusion. Aside from these little treasure tidbits, his shows always circle back to the digestive system.

TRIANGLE OF DISEASE

The part of his show I believe is tremendously important, and what I will use in this book to reference Landon's health, is what Ben calls the "triangle of disease": the three foundation points of all disease. This is a concept I find myself incessantly defaulting back to not only for Landon, but for myself, friends' and family's sake as well. I will continue to do so for the rest of my life. The triangle he outlines is an energy processing system comprised of the digestive system, the blood sugar area, and the adrenal thyroid complex. The body breaks down in this order at these three points. Each of the three points need to be functioning correctly in order to maintain a healthy system to stave off degenerative disease.

BREAKDOWN POINT ONE
- THE DIGESTIVE SYSTEM -

The first point of the triangle to break down, and the most discussed topic of all, is the digestive system. It is responsible for gathering energy. Gut Dysbiosis, or "messed up gut bacteria" begins for most of us at birth. Ben emphatically states this is the cause of any chronic degenerative disease, and speaks very often about the significance and the role of the gut. It is the most difficult part of the body to repair thus emphasizing the need to heal the gut with all the care and nurturing like you would give a baby. You can achieve this through proper foods, nutrition and supplementation. He mentioned wild fermented foods over and over, as well as organic bone soup, something which became a staple in my home later on. Bone soup, he said, contains collagen and many amino acids such as NAC (N-Acetylcysteine), hyaluronic acid and other minerals paramount to healing and sealing your digestive tract. Many additional supplements can be used to help this area as well, such as probiotics, zinc, and glutamine, to name a few. As far as diet is concerned, he is unwavering. Elimination of sugar, grains, pastas, breads, and especially alcohol are a must if you want to maintain a healthy digestive tract. (This may be difficult for me to handle.)

Usually Ben reserves the last 20 minutes of his show to callers who have health issue questions. Virtually all of them are met with the same question from Ben. "Do you have any digestive issues such as constipation, diarrhea, IBS, GERD, etc?" Every single one I have heard to this day has said yes. They all had digestive issues of some kind evidently linked to their ailment. His method was always about fixing the gut first in order to resolve the ailment. He made it clear no matter what health issue you have, you need to start at the digestive level and work from there.

BREAKDOWN POINT TWO
- BLOOD SUGAR -

The second breakdown point of the triangle is the blood sugar area, in charge of storing and releasing energy. If your doctor has told you have blood sugar issues, you have arrived. A sign your blood sugar may be out of whack is if it reads at very high or very low levels. Ben says the link between the digestive point and blood sugar point is probiotics, as well as creating an environment best suited for good bacteria to grow. If you do reach this blood sugar breakdown level, he recommends simple things you can do to regulate this point, such as using vitamin B complex, vitamin D, alpha lipoic acid, and magnesium. I do recall on one of his shows years earlier, Ben spoke about how the body flushes itself of magnesium when you have high blood sugar levels. It would only make sense to replenish yourself with magnesium that you lost. These are a few of the many ways he speaks of that aid in stabilizing blood sugar as well as blood pressure issues. People I know have done this and thrown away their medications. In addition to these blood sugar tips, Ben always emphasizes to make sure you move the body...sweat!

BREAKDOWN POINT THREE
– ADRENAL THYROID COMPLEX -

The third breakdown point of this triangle is the adrenal thyroid area, in charge of distributing energy. Hypothyroidism or what Ben calls the "jumping off" point, is where he says all chronic degenerative disease sets in. It is at this point you are in dire need to reverse course. To put it bluntly, if your thyroid is not up to par, you become susceptible to all disease. You do not want to reach this point of the triangle breakdown. Think of it as a red flag or flashing warning sign up ahead signaling that you are in great danger!

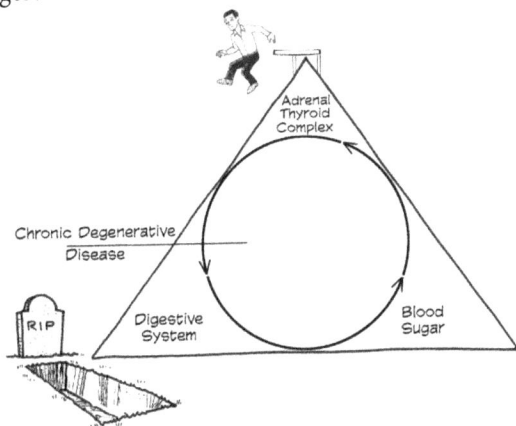

Each area is affected by the other in a constant cycle inside the triangle. If chronic degenerative disease does set in, you cannot just supplement at the level of the thyroid and hope your disease goes away. You need to go back to the base level and repair the digestive and blood sugar areas since they are interconnected. Ultimately, if you can maintain a healthy gut, you will be preventing thyroid and blood sugar breakdown at the same time. I recall several things you can do to assist the adrenal thyroid area. He often mentions calming the body down when it comes to this third point, through deep breathing exercises or anything that involves relaxation. I have heard him mention the majority of the population is unknowingly deficient in iodine, a critical element the thyroid needs to function properly in releasing hormones to the body. I also learned iodine was removed from regular table salt decades back, but can be found in mineral salts I mentioned earlier (Himalayan and Celtic sea salt). On several different shows I recall hearing how mineral salts contain essential elements of your body's makeup that are beneficial to the adrenals and thyroid. Selenium aids in thyroid function as well, and is one of the most referenced of all supplements on his show. These are just a few of the many notes I can remember. Knowing that a healthy thyroid is so vital to one's well-being, avoiding a thyroid disorder at all costs should be a standard objective.

Since Landon started off with a significantly impaired digestive system, he was way behind the curve. We came to find out later, he was right at the "jumping off point" (the degenerative disease level where all three points of his triangle were broken down) due to his leaky gut. The whole thing really made sense to me afterwards when I took a step back and looked. When we did test Landon's blood sugar that following day, it was dangerously low (Hypoglycemia), not high like I expected Sugar had been removed from his diet for the past few months, singled out by Ed and I as the main culprit of his distress. How we arrived at this reasoning comes into play later. We did not know what his low blood sugar reading meant at the time, or what to do. It was a catch 22 of sorts because it appeared giving him sugar presented serious consequences, and now it looks like prohibiting it also did as well. Landon had two of three points, the digestive and blood sugar, definitely breaking down and severely affected already. His thyroid condition remained to be seen. I did know that we were going to do everything we could to try and heal him at the digestive level and maybe this would start to balance things out. Breast milk, Ben says, is very important in the early stages to building the digestive tract. (I guess I screwed that up!) Although I did feel a little bit of relief for breastfeeding him the first several months, in my opinion it was a dire mistake to stop.

According to Ben, pharmaceutical drugs do not factor into the balance of this triangle, they only add to the toxicity. In fact, Ben often challenges doctors to come on his show if they disagree with his position on this or any topic at all. I have to agree with him about some of these medications. How many times do you see a prescription medication commercial where they tell you all the possible side effects? May cause heart attack, stroke, anaphylaxis, suicidal thoughts, death, etc. I don't know about you but to me it sounds like an acknowledgment that this is what will happen. When I am given a dire warning such as that, my first instinct is to run the other way. Always in support of supplementation, he makes a well founded argument when he says supplements or nutrients are used by the body, and prescription drugs are discarded.

I eventually got up enough nerve to call into the show and speak with Ben. We spoke about Landon's issues as well as questions I had relating to differences between methylcobalamin and cyanocobalamin, two forms of B12. He suggested many things we could do to start healing Landon but it would not be that easy. I told him almost everything at this point seemed intolerable to his gut, which made us afraid to even use supplements. The last thing I wanted to do was introduce anything new to his reactive immune system. Landon was in such pain every day it was difficult to figure out where one reaction ended and where one began since we constantly changed things up. Looking back, I would have taken swifter action with supplementation had I known there was no chance his body could have a reaction to essential vitamins. Ben nailed down specific vitamins and minerals we needed to start him on immediately, along with liquid probiotics, which would be more readily absorbed by his injured gut (great advice). I might add, Ben is also the spokesman for "Youngevity", a company selling many forms of health supplements that I have ordered from. One of the few supplements I bought for myself that he spoke about was a vitamin drink called Tangy Tangerine. For Landon this may have been too potent and too much to throw at him at once, so I held off for the time being.

After the successful and healthy birth of my third child, Cole, I began spending all my time on the internet trying to find answers to leaky gut. I found myself doggedly obsessed with this mystery. Pointed in the right direction, we needed to figure out how to fix this. If the doctors couldn't help us then we were going to get to the bottom of this ourselves. I knew deep inside, all these problems Landon was having must have something to do with the antibiotics and Prednisone (steroid for inflammation) prescribed for me during my pregnancy. I heard Ben speak of Prednisone once or twice and referred to it as poison and one of the most toxic of all drugs. I cringed as I recalled taking this multiple times while pregnant with Landon to treat a lung infection. Perhaps this was part of the whole gestalt that would be revealed soon enough.

BABYCENTER INTERVENTION

During another grueling week on the internet, and staunchly certain of my complicity to all of Landon's problems, I decided to cross reference eczema and antibiotics/Prednisone. Little did I know this one post would be so life changing. BINGO! I had finally hit upon a bombshell, possibly a big piece of the puzzle. On a

BabyCenter (www.babycenter.com) forum, of all places, was a woman named Kerri, telling a story, one very similar to ours. As I read on, I could not take my eyes off of what I was reading. I was thunderstruck. It was like I was reading my own narrative! Her compelling story started off by telling the world about her son and his eczema. She described his problems, and they were all the identical problems Landon was having. She sat up nights praying to find an answer as to why her son was scratching himself to death, why he was allergic to everything, and how he was becoming neurologically impaired. Her story was indistinguishable to ours, and this site was the godsend we were looking for. She explained how she researched the library for answers and came across a book by Dr. Kenneth Bock, MD called "Healing the New Childhood Epidemics: Autism, ADHD, Asthma, and Allergies: The Groundbreaking Program for the 4-A Disorders."[3] He wrote about how the gut impacts disorders such as ADHD, Allergies, Autism and Asthma and described his groundbreaking program to heal these disorders. (Aha! A doctor who knows something!) As Kerri relayed her story on this forum, she revealed that her child had had an internal yeast infection! After reading Bock's book she realized it was the yeast that was the main cause of most of these problems. She disclosed if you've ever given your child antibiotics or Prednisone like she had, a yeast overgrowth can occur causing numerous intestinal problems, such as eczema and allergies, and ultimately developmental disorders. She knew her son needed antifungals.

Of course! I was given antibiotics and prednisone during pregnancy. This was an almost identical situation to ours, and what she was saying made sense to me. The problem is, I've never heard of a doctor prescribing an antifungal for a child. I always assumed they were for women with vaginal yeast infections. Would they prescribe this if you asked them? Would a doctor agree to this if they did not come up with the diagnosis on their own? Now you may say to yourself, "What's the problem? Just go to your friendly local pediatrician and ask for a prescription for an antifungal." It's not that easy! She was able to acquire the antifungal from her pediatrician when she came to the doctor appointment armed with Dr. Bock's book. I was not so sure about our pediatrician. I know enough about doctors, judges, and lawyers to say that people in those professions do not like being told how to do their job by the average Jane. If you were in a courtroom on the stand, daring to cite the law to a judge, he would find a reason to throw the book at you. Walking in the doctor's office demanding or even requesting a prescription for Diflucan for a child would most likely be a mistake. We needed to approach this strategically.

Kerri also gave an alternative solution in case your pediatrician chose not to prescribe an antifungal. She said DAN doctors (An organization called "Defeat Autism Now," now named ARI "Autism Research Institute", also referred to as "Biomedical" doctors) are what you may want to look for. She explained these types of doctors use modern medicine along with nutritional therapies and more than likely will know if your child has yeast issues. They would also be more likely to prescribe an antifungal if this was the case. Since then I noticed the labels of these doctors fluctuate even though they apply the same or similar practice. Over time I have seen the label change from biomedical, to integrative medicine, to MAPS, to functional medicine. This struck me as a little odd, having to make an appointment with an autism doctor, unless…I erased the thought from my mind only to have it come rushing back. Could Landon be autistic? Is this a link? Kerri went on to say she healed her son. Once she resolved his yeast issues, which required months of antifungals, the allergies went away and his behavior returned to normal. Undoubtedly, this woman was exceptionally intuitive. She actually had the intuition to foresee possible roadblocks that may arise with the pediatricians and devised a game plan for everyone just in case. It was much later I realized just how far ahead of the game she put us. For the time being, this was the least of my concerns. All I cared about at that moment was this revelation she gifted, and the desire to get a move on. I could barely contain myself and counted the minutes before Ed returned home and I could give him the news. He was skeptical to say the least and doubtful this was going to provide us with any different results. In that moment, I could not have been more thrilled had I discovered a cure for cancer.

I ordered Dr. Bock's book and in the meantime, I voraciously began reading up about yeast/candida. Countless hours were spent researching articles and studies regarding yeast and disease. I was certain not only was Landon's digestive tract consumed, his blood was infected with it. We needed to cleanse his blood and his body.

ELAINE AND DYLAN

An important day in our journey was meeting a woman name Elaine and her son Dylan at the local library. While we described to her Landon's eczema, allergies, and intestinal issues, she stared at us with eyes wide open. Her son had had the same exact issues as Landon, starting at birth. He was three and a half now but she described to us in duplicate detail the long nights of terror as he screamed in pain, back arched, allergic to everything! As an infant, his skin had the same weeping eczema as Landon had. And there was one more thing: she also had taken prednisone during pregnancy for a poison ivy outbreak! I was now convinced there had to be a correlation with this drug and these problems. We dissected our stories and began putting the pieces together. We had each taken prednisone and both Landon and Dylan exhibited the same complications. I tried quickly explaining to her about yeast and the forum I discovered, but seemed to get lost more in my quest for answers from her.

It felt like a one in a million encounter. Then I thought more about the odds of that chance encounter. Since I do not believe in coincidences, I came to a different conclusion. Maybe it was not such a long shot we encountered each other, maybe this was widespread. Just how many other women has this happened to as well? Someone needs to sound the alarm. We commiserated about our feelings of helplessness as we watched the same horror play out night after night and day after day right before our eyes as we searched for answers. Like us, she had carried Dylan around 24/7, and he would not let her put him down. He also had the same anaphylactic reaction to peanuts as Landon, and would vomit most other foods. Basically, he was allergic to almost everything, just like Landon. Now at age 3, he had overcome a lot of those allergies and could even eat a burger. Maybe there was hope, but what did they do different to conquer these hurdles? Looking back, I believe giving Landon formula (I explain in the next few chapters) had a lot to do with the differences, as well as something else which presented itself later.

As we talked, I watched Dylan as he played and interacted. He was a very polite, perfectly adjusted little boy. Elaine called Dylan over to introduce us. He walked over and said hi to us with a smile, then scurried off to play with another little girl. We watched amusingly as he imitated He-Man, flexing his arms as they both giggled. I was overjoyed to see her son had overcome these issues and turned out the way he had. I looked over at Landon and one noticeable difference was his bloated tummy. Elaine told us Dylan's stomach was always concave, never swollen or bloated. His weight gain problem however was the same. We asked many questions about how and when the change occurred and what she did to help him.

One main difference we discovered was that Elaine breastfed for two years. She had spent years eating only what her son could tolerate, meanwhile denying herself the nutritious benefits of foods such as eggs, meats, and healthy fats such as butter. Since Dylan was allergic to all of this, she did not eat any of it. She explained how she suffered, as her hair began falling out and her skin turned very dry. I commended her for doing this and secretly chastised myself for stopping so soon. I knew it was the best thing for Landon, but did not grasp just how important it was.

An incident I will share that weighs heavily on my mind was a definite contributing factor as to why I prematurely stopped breastfeeding. I know now it was a pea-brained decision, but I accepted a challenge (more arrogance on my part) as an incentive to lose more baby weight. Since I never back down from a physical challenge, I agreed to race an NHL player down the length of an ice rink skating forwards while he skated backwards. Most of these NHL players can skate faster backwards than most people can forwards, but I did not believe he stood a chance. I asked for one month to get in hard core shape. Prior to this, I decided to start shedding weight, and by the time the skate-off arrived, I dropped a total of 30 pounds. This is what most likely caused my lactation to slow down considerably, which made it easy to convince myself to stop breastfeeding. In retrospect, I see what a disadvantage I put Landon at. The repercussions only occurred to me years later when I dissected all the possibilities associated with Landon's health issues. Even if I am wrong and this had little to do with anything, it certainly did not help matters. Ultimately Elaine and Dylan were both survivors. We could only hope in a few years, things would look up for Landon.

GMO GOOD? OMG!

Outside of the doctor's office, we had nowhere to turn for information. Because my father is a professional in the dental field, a pathologist, I decided to approach him, and discuss this yeast/Leaky Gut theory with him. As quickly as I was able to broach the question, he was able to abruptly shut me down. What a mistake this was. Without even hearing me out, I had to listen to him insult me about how I could not possibly know what I'm talking about because I do not have a medical degree. Funny, because I felt as if I gained more knowledge in the previous year than many of those geniuses who saw Landon, would ever know. Apparently, Leaky Gut was a term he had never heard before, therefore anything I said subsequent to this was disregarded. There was one thing I was certain of in my mind. Dr. Bock, who went to medical school, and Ben Fuchs, whose knowledge in my opinion surpassed many of the doctors I had met, do know what they are talking about. At that time, they were the only ones making sense to me, but neither was there to speak for me.

On another occasion I had tried to explain my fears about genetically modified food to my father, and how all we could give Landon was organic food. Surprisingly, he had not heard of GMO and asked "what does GMO stand for?" Even though he obviously was not educated on the subject, he defensively attacked my credibility, indicating again that I was someone with no medical training, and had no business speaking with authority to him about anything with the words "genetic" in them. Genetically modified is good for us, he said. After hearing this, I could only conclude that the words "genetic" and "modified" resulted in a conclusion in his mind that GMO has to be better for us because it involves DNA, science, and labs. An observant person would be able to see the food today is not what it used to be. Something has changed, making it much less tolerable on the gut. Looking at grocery store food labels would be a more common sense approach. Even some of the most well known food companies go out of their way to label their food "Non-GMO". If GMO was a positive breakthrough, wouldn't they be labeling it "contains GMO"? Like other medical professionals we had encountered, my father was not open to new information, and instead resorted to personal disparagement and verbal abuse rather than engaging in a discussion. I noticed this was a common tactic he often used with most guests in his house as it was the easiest and quickest way to silence the opposition and be declared the winner. If that did not work, a tantrum would be thrown and the guest would be told to leave his house. He was obviously too defensive about the time and money he had spent studying medicine, to consider that there could be new breakthroughs in alternative medicines that might make it to mainstream one day. This really left me with nobody to discuss health topics with in my immediate family.

In my mind, there had to be some value to all of the shared experiences we were encountering: Why was everyone so quick to dismiss unpopular paths of action? What was clear now was that all conversations about this or any matter with my father were done; he had closed the door on any future discussions. We were on our own.

3

OH MY CANDIDA

My new obsession now turned to autism and candida. Our guess at this stage of the journey was that Landon's broken metabolism and leaky gut was linked to this Candida problem. Based on all the reading I have done, yeast, in my opinion, is the most vile, wretched, repulsive organism in existence. I believe wholeheartedly it is behind every disease known to man. Men, you need to let go of the misconception that yeast is a women's issue. You are not exempt. If you have taken heavy rounds of antibiotics/oral steroids, consume a diet consisting of substantial amounts of sugar and alcohol, then my guess is you are probably loaded with it. All of these combined may qualify you as a walking brewery. Yeast does not discriminate! I began searching the internet for autism signs and symptoms, and its relation to Candida. Ei-resource.org had an article called "The Candida Yeast-Autism Connection" by Stephen M. Edelson, Ph.D Center for the Study of Autism. He writes, "There is a great deal of evidence that a form of yeast, Candida albicans, may cause autism and may exacerbate many behaviors and health problems in autistic individuals, especially those with late-onset autism."[4] His next paragraph tied in antibiotics. "Candida albicans belongs to the yeast family and is a single-cell fungus. This form of yeast is located in various parts of the body including the digestive tract."[5] He speaks about benign microbes keeping the yeast under control. "However, exposure to antibiotics, especially repeated exposure, can destroy these microbes. This can result in an overgrowth of Candida albicans. When the yeast multiplies, it releases toxins in the body; and these toxins are known to impair the central nervous system and the immune system."[6]

Landon was showing many signs of autism, but I was still in denial because he had eye contact and could smile. However, this meant nothing because there is what is called an "autism spectrum". Along the spectrum you will see kids on the extreme low-functioning end, to ones all the way on the high functioning end. Landon functioned so I did not know if this meant he was on the spectrum. He exhibited autistic symptoms but did this mean he was autistic? Next, the article states the problems that manifest from candida overgrowth. "Confusion, hyperactivity, short attention span, lethargy, irritability, and aggression. Health problems can include: headaches, stomachaches, constipation, gas pains, fatigue, and depression."[7] Treating candida was mentioned as well which required supplements and medication. "Taking nutritional supplements which replenish the intestinal tract with good microbes (e.g., acidophilus) and/or taking anti-fungal medications (Nystatin, Ketoconosal, Diflucan). It is also recommended that the person be placed on a special diet low in sugar on which yeasts thrive."[8]

A horrible feeling came over me. Landon had been on that baby formula for well over a year. The nutritional information on the back of the formula container indicated there was a high content of sugar. If sugar feeds yeast, and Landon did have an internal yeast infection, then the sugar we were feeding him on a daily basis was rapidly causing the yeast to multiply. We had to get him off that formula and find an alternative nutrient source!

The next part I read was similar to what Kerri had spoken about in the BabyCenter forum: "If the Candida albicans is causing health and behavior problems, a person will often become quite ill for a few days after receiving a treatment to kill the excess yeast. The yeast is destroyed and the debris is circulated through the body until it is excreted. Thus, a person who displays negative behaviors soon after receiving treatment for candida (Herxheimer reaction) is likely to have a good prognosis."[9] Kerri strongly emphasized that her son had the Herxheimer reaction or what she called a "die off" for quite awhile. His behavior became worse until he excreted the yeast through his bowels, and then he improved a little bit at a time after each die-off. She made sure to mention her son had to remain on antifungals for months at a time or there would be a possibility for the yeast to grow back. The spores needed to be killed off. Edelson notes "treatment for candida infrequently results in a cure for autism. However, if the person is suffering from this problem, his/her health and behavior should improve following the therapy."[10]

After reading many articles similar to this one, some confusion clouded our minds. Questions in my mind plagued me as I struggled to find answers to them. Was Landon autistic or did he just have Candida? If his yeast is a common denominator associated with autism, and he has displayed a lot of other similar symptoms, then does that mean he is autistic? Did these yeast/digestive issues cause autism or do autistic kids just have them in common? Reading all this was hard for me, and especially Ed, to grasp. Ed couldn't fathom Landon was autistic. He correlated the word autistic with a child who is just not there, one in his/her own little world oblivious to the real world. I also did not want to believe it, and was reading everything and anything to convince myself these problems will pass, and he will outgrow it. Even though we had been denying to this point that Landon was autistic, he had all the same digestive issues an autistic child has and some behavioral ones as well.

Christmas that year was meaningless. Landon did not have the capacity to experience joy from opening presents, and he spent most of the time incessantly crying. Besides the titanic meltdowns, other scary signs he began showing included OCD behaviors, head banging, excessive drooling, word and sound repetition, night-time hyperactivity, super silly behavior, bloated stomach, and dark circles under his eyes (allergies). He could hardly eat any foods, and the foods he could eat were not supplying nutrients to his body. Time seemed to be running out and Landon's weight continued to drop with each passing day. I called the pediatrician's office the following business day to make an appointment, meanwhile formulating a plan on how to cajole his doctor for a three month prescription of Diflucan. (Interesting to note, it did not even occur to us we had natural options available.) If this did not work, it would have to be plan B, a biomedical intervention the mothers on BabyCenter spoke about.

Meanwhile, I read Dr. Bock's book twice from beginning to end. His book was way more involved (and technical) than candida, and I knew if Landon's issue wasn't resolved from antifungals then we had a much bigger problem on our hands. The book also contained deeply sincere and emotional stories about the many children he has helped heal over the years. I have probably given away three copies of his book to other parents since first reading it, for its informational value alone. After finishing the book, I thought to myself, all I have to do is march into the pediatrician's office the next day with this book, explain the problem, and ask him nicely for a prescription for Diflucan.

The day finally arrived. As I drove Landon to the appointment, I prepared myself for that "crazy mom alert" reaction from the doctor those moms in BabyCenter warned me about. Sure enough, he looked at my three heads and eight arms as he mentally constructed a mile high wall between us I knew would be next to impossible to climb over. Book in hand, I showed him the chapters about Candida and how Landon's symptoms and health decline match consistently to symptoms of yeast overgrowth. I believe this is what is referred to as stepping on someone's toes. Out of spite alone from being lectured about medicine, his answer was an emphatic no. After five minutes of accosting him with information in Bock's book, his only objective was the door and how to get it open, and get me out of that office as quickly as possible. Irritated by his ignorance, I tried three different occasions with this same office hoping a different doctor would give me a different response. None of them wanted to cooperate. Not one would even entertain the idea, and all acted as if I was insulting their expertise. In fact, I was being treated like there was something wrong with me! Kerri must have had some mad negotiating skills that I just did not possess. Most likely, I was not delicate in my delivery. Time was closing in, and I did not have time to be delicate or worry about disrespecting someone's feelings. Down but not out, I realized I was probably now flagged in the system as a nuisance, so I decided to move on.

Many questions remain unanswered. Why did none of these doctors we spoke to even want to consider this as a cause or a problem, even after I showed them possible evidence of other cases? How do you make six figures a year in the medical field, and not understand yeast or Leaky Gut Syndrome? Did Dr. Bock have a broader reach of certain information that these doctors do not have access to? Did he attend a medical school of higher learning? If yeast was the case with Landon, (and I was certain it was at this point) I can only imagine the dreadful effects it had on Landon as a developing fetus and the continued effect it was still having. I felt as if the doctors' treatments were to try every possible symptom relieving medicine, while never considering the cause. I'm surprised I was not given a phony name for a rare condition Landon had such as "Bellibloatitis Inflamarxinomous". Most people would most likely consent to this diagnosis as make believe as it is! In my opinion, too much power is put into the doctors' hands because a typical parent would accept a doctor's word at face value. What if they are wrong? Walking out that day, I was done with these doctors. As far as I was concerned these pediatricians should have their medical licenses stripped and not be allowed to return until they go back to school and actually learn something, anything. If not beginner's biology, what kind of curriculum were they being taught? Why did I have to beg them to do their job? We were obviously looking for help in all the wrong places.

When we returned home, I went back to the BabyCenter website with Kerri and read through the thread, hoping each time I could get something new from it. Believing that these moms were onto something valid, I sought for more backup information. I searched and found another Candida thread just as beneficial. This was like a sort of secret society of Candida moms, and it was a beautiful thing. It was like they existed outside the realm of mainstream all banding together in support of one another and their children's yeast issues. I was appalled what a scary pandemic this was really turning out to be. I must have spent the next three weeks on those threads (which were still going strong last time I checked). I was also hoping there were other cases out there I had not seen before. I concluded I needed to get our hands on an antifungal prescription, and in order to do this, I knew I had to find a doctor who knew about yeast: a DAN or Biomedical Doctor.

I increasingly believed autism was a strong possibility. Autism or not, I believed a biomedical doctor could at least treat him for yeast and help us in that area. In my mind, the main culprit had to be yeast. Trying to wrap our heads around this debacle felt very foreign. Just like the article mentioned earlier, Bock explained in many chapters how sugar feeds yeast which thus grows exponentially when it is fed. The yeast then pokes holes in the digestive tract. Once the damage has occurred, it gets worse as you feed it and the body becomes dysfunctional in a multitude of ways. He calls this intestinal hyperpermeability, aka leaky gut syndrome. These serious problems due to yeast overgrowth he calls "fungal dysbiosis."[11] I recall Ben and Bock mentioning other variables such as parasites or alcohol may also cause leaky gut, but in our case, evidence suggested to us it was yeast. What we were now learning made complete sense to me, and apparently to other parents as well. It confounded me that these conditions related to the immune system that had unheard of roots of origin along with unfamiliar remedies, were working for people and were not more publicized.

This is why diet later became the most important catalyst in our education. We had fed Landon sugar laden baby formula for such a long time and I was certain it had been a major contributor to the yeast overgrowth. Whether he had other issues to go along with this was a question mark. Landon seemed to be progressing at times, but I knew we needed to stop accepting his slow development as normal.

Worst case scenario was that I would call Dr. Bock and make an appointment with him in Red Hook NY. Before I did this, I wanted to investigate closer options. I looked online for a bio-medical doctor in Connecticut and found one close by. There were only two or three in the entire state, which told us some-thing. Either not many doctors are educated about Candida and biomedical science, or this is just all a bunch of horse manure! We later learned a lot of these biomedical doctors all had person-al experiences with autism and chose this field for that reason. They perhaps knew something other doctors did not.

One question that kept popping up in my mind was why were none of these parents of autistic children being told there are oth-er alternative things they can try? Even my parents, who follow mainstream medicine, insisted that Landon's case was a behavior-al issue (I talk about this later on) and we are raising a spoiled child whom we cater to 24/7. We had been under attack from my parents for some time about why were we not vaccinating this child, and how we cannot ignore the science behind vaccines. When I say attack, I speak lightly. It was a daily bombardment of unrelenting verbal assaults and they would not let up. Any chance they got was used as an attempt to assassinate our character and call us irresponsible neglectful parents. I soon became sick and tired of this. After about three months, Ed and I told them they were not allowed in our house anymore if they cannot accept our decisions and support us regardless of whether they agree with us or not. It was the beginning of what was to become a long ex-tended feud in our family, and would usually result in someone being thrown out of the house. We felt pushed to the edge. Tired of trying to explain to them about our beliefs behind this, we de-cided it was better off to keep our distance. Just like the saying goes, "If you don't stand for something, you will fall for anything." We didn't live for them or anybody, and most definitely were nev-er ones for "go along to get along". We did, however, know who we were and what we stood for. This relates back to the first quote in chapter one, "know who you are." It was simply our opinions and we were holding our ground.

Because I did not hold an MD, I held no persuasive abilities to my family. Nobody wanted to listen. I want to specify again that not vaccinating was our personal choice, and the last thing I'm going to do is change my mind for somebody else because the 6 o'clock news ran a story suggesting it's the responsible thing to do. This was literally the case here. Married to the 6 o'clock news, my parents' advice, judgment, and information they cast our way was regurgitated from a credible sounding news anchor wearing a suit and tie. Credible to them meant well dressed and Ivy League educated. I do not get my facts from the 6 o'clock news, and will not be told what to think, regardless of the news anchor's Harvard education. Nevertheless, vaccines have little to do with this story and nothing to do with our son having autism so there really is no argument here, it does not even apply. One of the factors behind our decision not to vaccinate was simply reading. Well meaning people suggested, if we have questions, just go to the CDC website or ask the doctor if you could read the inserts. If an insert reads "can cause measles, measles like rash, diabetes, encephalitis, Guillain-Barre syndrome, pneumonia and even death," I am surely not going to let a doctor inject my vulnerable child with the possibility of any of this occurring. If the disease itself is a side effect of what I am trying to prevent, I'm going to think twice. Basically, we did not want to inject anything into our son's already weakened immune system that has not matured, especially with the possibility of one of those side effects. It just did not make sense to us. Also, if any of those side effects were to occur there's no liability for the vaccine makers. Why would I feel their vaccine is safe to inject if they cannot even back up its safety?

On a comical side note, I recall hearing about a million dollar vaccine challenge presented to thousands of vaccine company executives, by two radio hosts (Mike Adams the Health Ranger & Alex Jones). Alex declared that what is most injurious are the adjuvants within the vaccines. Intent on proving to listeners their stance regarding harmful side effects of vaccines, they dared these vaccine makers and executives to validate the safety of the vaccines they stood behind. Hence, Mike and Alex propositioned them to take one thousand of their own shots, at one thousand dollars per shot, over a two week period (500 Influenza shots, 100 Anthrax shots, 100 Polio shots, 100 Gardasil shots, 100 Hepatitis B shots, 100 Meningitis shots). Considering the promoters' stance that any number of vaccines can be safely received by a child, I believed this challenge would not only be accepted but also theoretically been a cakewalk for an adult. Vaccine advocate Piers Morgan was additionally given the same one million dollar challenge. This no longer sounded funny to me when I learned neither Piers nor the executives came forward to accept the challenge. As amusing as this dare was, the lack of response is something to take into consideration upon drawing your own conclusion.

Getting bullied by local pediatricians made us fight harder. I apologize to them if I perhaps thwarted their opportunity for a large yearend bonus from the insurers' "Performance Recognition Program", for not letting them vaccinate my child. My opinion about this is as follows: once you move forward, there is no turning back the clock. You may not only get blamed for some of those side effects, but in the end, nobody except you is left to pick up the pieces. We know there is a lot of contention about vaccines causing autism, but again, it did not pertain to us. I wrote this to support why we came to the conclusions we did.

On the other hand, many people believe that vaccines are a big factor and if you vaccinate an unhealthy child, this may be a big component to what causes autism. I personally know nurses who will not vaccinate their own children under any circumstances. One in particular told me she has seen enough to know better. After seeing how ill Landon was, even one of our doctors later said to us as we left the office, "If you vaccinate him, you will lose him." We were not being told anything we did not already inherently feel. Even though we already kind of lost part of Landon, in our opinion, we felt vaccinating him may have brought him to a point of no return. I feel it would have been a grave mistake to vaccinate him in the vulnerable state he was in. I spoke to some parents who said their child developed neurological tics, seizures and never regained language. One mother from Greece whom I met in Florida told me her son was fine until the day after he got his MMR. He awoke the next morning after the vaccination, unable to speak like before and was never the same. I was invited over their house by her oldest son one day for dinner and met their lovely family. Her youngest son was now 24, but had the language of a 3 year old, fixated mostly on objects and little tasks. Having no receptive language, he could not listen to explanations or instructions, and would randomly make statements that did not relate to the conversation at hand. She told me flat out, the MMR vaccine caused his autism. She is not the only parent to be certain of this cause and outcome. Better safe than sorry!

Dr. Bock explains in his book that autism is caused by metabolic dysfunction and toxicity. With vaccines being ruled out by us as the cause of toxicity, it did not mean Landon was not loaded with toxins (most likely from me). Whatever it happened to be, Landon was losing cognitive ability and regressing on a weekly basis.

4

BIOMEDICAL TREATMENT BEGINS

The appointment with our first biomedical doctor was with a woman I will call Dr. C. The visit lasted 2-½ hours and the cost was extensive. Everything was out of pocket including the cost of the appointment itself, the blood draw, and the supplements. Before bringing Landon in for his first appointment with this doctor, I had plan B already implemented to start him on natural antifungals in case we were not prescribed the medical grade kind. During the examination, Landon's screams could be heard throughout the building. Her reaction alone was convincing enough to me that we were out of our league. As Landon had his exorcism fit, Dr. C urgently rushed down the hallway shouting instructions to her staff to help her. She seemed reserved to tell us, but we could read between the lines. His issues went much deeper than yeast alone.

Our primary goal in coming here was to get antifungals because in our mind his only issue was yeast. We never asked her the question and she never said the word either. We all ignored the big elephant in the room...is Landon autistic? I believe we did not ask because we still thought maybe this could be resolved with Diflucan. Secondly, we did not want to know. I can only speculate she did not bring it up because she did not want us to kill the messenger. I'm sure a lot of parents would take offense to a doctor telling them their child is autistic, especially those in denial. She threw a list of a dozen tasks we needed to get started on right away. Abrasively and without explanation, she conveyed it would require immediate action. Her unkind manner alone scared us and I believe it was this fear we had of her that made us feel apprehensive about continuing on. We came there hungry for knowledge yet felt as if her answers were more like reprimands for having the gall to ask questions.

After one seemingly innocent question, she looked up from her notes exasperated and began lecturing us that she had been doing this for 20+ years; in other words, "zip it". Funny thing is, none of our questions were attacks on her. Our questions served a purpose and mainly were asked out of a deep curiosity about Landon's condition. Instead of feeling attacked, she should have felt flattered we had come to her for answers. She made clear none of the things he was doing were normal; spinning in circles, repetitive word syllables, walking like a drunken sailor, screaming, and digestive agony. She explained his drunk like behavior or impaired walking was due to the neurotoxin acetaldehyde, which is a by-product of the yeast.

She listed in her report encephalitis of the brain (swelling). I wasn't so sure about swelling of the brain. If that were the case, wouldn't he be in the same condition all the time? He did have moments where he seemed calm and undisturbed. I never did accept that as part of the diagnosis, I treated it as more of an assumption on her part. She immediately put him on probiotics (PB 8, Theralac) to re-establish gut flora that the antibiotics wiped out and went over a diet plan as well. I mentioned to her that Landon developed a rash/allergic reaction from the probiotics we were already giving him. In a tone rather unbecoming, she got in my face and clamored, "That's die-off!". Translation: it's die-off you idiot. We did not know probiotics were strong enough to cause die-off, but in the grand scheme of things, it makes sense. After this verbal transaction, we moved onto diet. She told us no more salmon or trout that we had been feeding him due to the high toxicity levels. She suggested lamb or turkey to which he never reacted to and still eats today. She explained Landon's weight loss. Since Landon's intestinal tract was out of whack, he could not absorb nutrients from food. He looked very sickly now with the dark circles under the eyes and a protruding belly. He needed supplements due to the malabsorption issue. She prescribed these indefinitely until his digestive tract was healthy enough to digest and metabolize food. She handed us a blood, stool and urine collection kit which contained 12 blood collection tubes, as well as lab orders for the things she would be testing. (Allergies, IGG/ IGE, heavy metals, vitamin and mineral deficiencies, etc.) Twelve tubes of blood from a two-year-old? I was not sure he had that much blood flowing inside him. How were we going to even get through the blood draw without him setting off an emergency broadcast alert?

As this question weighed in the back of our minds, we also had to deal with the barrage of supplements we needed to start him on. How would he react to them? Will I remember what to give him, when to give it to him, and just how long will we have to do this? The supplements she gave us included vitamin C, vitamin E, a vitamin B12 (methylcobalamin) injection prescription to be ordered from a compounding pharmacy, zinc, GABA, cod liver oil, and taurine. "What about antifungals?", I asked. She responded, "antifungals come later". Later?! What the...? Someone needed to explain to me how this can wait. If a cut is infected, wouldn't you clean the infected area first before applying treatment? If you ask me, this is the same exact thing. Clean him out first, then supplement. I would have bet my life Landon had what I suspected; a massive internal yeast infection which I know could potentially kill him, or at the very least shut organs down if we wait. The neurological impact alone should be reason enough not to delay. This was the only reason we came here, to get the antifungal prescription! In my opinion, the first course of action should be to eliminate the cause of his leaky gut. It made zero sense to me why we would start supplements before eliminating the main source of the problem.

Not only were we denied the prescription, she began overwhelming us with scary stuff like needles and injections! Suddenly I came to a very unsettling realization as I mentally prepared myself for the unthinkable. I may become the first woman you read about in the news to get arrested for breaking and entering a Walgreens...to steal their supply of Diflucan. Just give it to us and we can be on our way! All this effort, and still we cannot even get a biomedical doctor to prescribe an antifungal, something I was certain in my soul would at least help resolve our problem overall. I theorized about reasons why she did not do this. Maybe she was worried we may quit the program after experiencing that savage die-off reaction we had read so much about? Or was it possible she wanted to dangle that carrot in front of us so we would have to keep coming back? Or antifungals really did come later in the program and perhaps we just needed to shut up and listen. As stubborn as I am, equipped with the knowledge I possessed, that would not be the case. Our decision now would be natural antifungals, something we kicked ourselves for not considering earlier.

During this time, I took the forum moms' advice and decided to read Jenny McCarthy's book "Louder than Words"[12], which relates her experiences with autism. I wish she had written five more chapters about this subject; I know I could have written an entire library about it. I cannot emphasize enough how incredibly important I think the topic of yeast and yeast die-off is, so I am about to tell you all about it in the next few chapters. We tried our best to prepare ourselves for what was about to take place. It is my belief that no parent can ever truly be prepared for this next step. In the world of parents with autistic children, crashing through the yeast barrier is what I consider a "rite of passage". I believe hundreds of thousands more could benefit from learning about what to expect from die-off, as well as the importance of how to survive the raging waters as you try to cross the river. The die-off reaction Jenny witnessed her son experience was similar to what the mothers on the BabyCenter forum spoke about, but much more extreme in her case. With this inevitable certainty looming over our heads, we prepared to buckle down.

5

MAN ON FIRE SYNDROME/
COCONUT KEFIR

For many weeks now I had been reading all about anti-fungals and how they cause what's called a "die-off" or "Herxheimer" reaction where the yeast gets killed quickly and overloads the body with toxins when they die. Dr. Jill Carnahan wrote an article called "Tips for Dealing with Herx-heimer or Die-off Reactions."[13] She talks about everything associated with yeast overgrowth such as leaky gut, antibiotic use, lack of good probiotics, and Herxheimer. If the toxins are not eliminated from the body quickly, the die-off can cause reactions including fever, chills, flu like symptoms, and extreme irritability. In our case it was overwhelming and terrifying for us to witness. I later came up with the term "man on fire syndrome.

Since we lost the battle of the prescription antifungals with the doctors, I researched natural ways to do this ourselves. Even though the yeast was largely conjecture on our part, Landon's lab work showed high yeast content in his urine analysis, which confirmed what we suspected from the beginning. Our goal was to rid him of the candida, balance his flora, and work to repair his gut lining. Along with the antifungal search, I also looked up more about Dr. Bock online. I came across a YouTube video with Dr. Bock, a child patient, and her parent getting interviewed on Fox News.

The parent was saying how coconut kefir reversed his daughter's autism. Coconut kefir? I had to look this up and find out what it was. Normally, I would have identified this as some kind of gimmick, especially after learning this man started his own coconut kefir business. After realizing he did this because of the effects it had on his daughter's condition, it made sense. Regardless, I knew by watching and listening to this man that he was being unconditionally sincere. Strange as this sounds, I remember I had a bottle of this in my fridge! I had bought it a few weeks earlier while searching for a probiotic for myself. It was a nondairy fermented coconut water probiotic made from young green coconuts. I bought it for myself because I was learning how unhealthy I was while in the process of doing all this research about Landon. I came to believe I was toxic during pregnancy and transferred all those bad toxins and candida over to Landon. Purchasing it for him to use was not intended, rather, I saw it more as a happy accident. After seeing this video, I ran and grabbed it from the fridge, excited and extremely hopeful we were onto something. That night I perused the entire internet about what coconut kefir is and the magic it can do for the body. Naturalnews.com had many articles, including one by David Jockers called "Discover the Superfood Power of Kefir"[14] explaining the benefits of kefir "recolonizing the gut with beneficial strains of microflora".[15] Other contributing articles I read were from draxe.com "Coconut Kefir: The Probiotic Food that Improves Immunity & Digestion"[16], bodyecology.com "2 Simple Steps to Detox Mercury and Other Heavy Metals"[17], and another called "How Cleansing Plays a Major Role in Autism Recovery."[18] All these articles speak highly of the effects of kefir as it cleanses the endocrine system, detoxes heavy metals, kills candida, brings the body's pH to an alkaline level, and supplies the body with essential minerals such as magnesium, lauric acid, biotin, vitamin K2, folate, enzymes and B vitamins.

This fountain of youth discovery would be incorporated as a mainstay of our everyday lives. Something this beneficial cannot be ignored. What I found ironic is that kefir is an antifungal that kills candida, a bad form of yeast, yet the kefir itself is a good type of yeast. It is what many agree to be the top tier of probiotics. According to Derek Henry's naturalnews article "The Healing Power of Coconut Kefir", he believes kefir stands alone as "the most healing and beneficial probiotic beverage."[19] We would learn this soon enough.

Our preparedness for what was to follow was about to pay off. We started Landon off with a half teaspoon twice a day in his hemp milk. We hoped he would not have a Herxheimer reaction, which would make this phase of the treatment very easy. Contrary to this delusion, two or three days after giving Landon this probiotic, all hell broke loose. Let me describe our harrowing ordeal with kefir.

Picture a person on fire, running and moving around trying to put out the flames, as they scream from the torture. We were hoping small amounts would be fine and not cause a major reaction, but we were wrong. What began as hair-raising cries of terror turned into a 24/7 ordeal of a psychotic screaming, kicking, biting, head banging nightmare. During these fits Landon would spit up white gooey excrement that had a wretched, vile smell. The itching would intensify and seem to get worse as his skin would weep in certain areas. At times he would have bouts of uncontrolled maniacal laughing, and other times his eyes would roll back in his head and he'd scream bloody murder as if being stabbed. We would be lying if we told you the word "institutionalized" never entered our minds. But the saving grace to us was the fact he was having a reaction at all meant we were on the right path. Like Jenny McCarthy said, it really did resemble a real life exorcism of sorts. (A fleeting thought entered my mind that maybe exorcisms are just people having a yeast die-off.)

The inappropriate laughter frightened me considerably. A friend of ours came by one day to pick up her daughter who was friends with my oldest daughter, Angela. As we stood around talking, Landon began a bout of uncontrollable laughter as he stood directly in front of her. It began out of nowhere without instigation from anyone. We passed it off as humorous until it happened again the next week she came over. Suddenly it was not funny anymore. We saw this before starting the kefir as well but it became more noticeable during this time period. In my opinion it was a sign of something worse to come.

The first time after seeing these reactions we stopped our kefir treatment cold turkey. However, after reading about reactions being a good sign not bad, we continued at lower doses. We frequently tried backing off and reducing the amount of kefir, and then tried building back up slowly. Each time, the die-off became too much for us to handle, let alone Landon. What kept me going and urging Ed to push forward was reading the sites and books that explain the die-off or Herxheimer reaction Edelson had described. Everything appeared as if the condition was getting worse and the child was regressing, however, if they are healing, he/she slowly progresses like a pendulum swinging them to a positive milestone. The man-on-fire syndrome would occur two or three times a day, only to have us jump ship at least a dozen times. This went on for so long I started to doubt it was a Herxheimer anymore due to the fact it should only last several days to weeks. I believed it to be more of a cleansing or healing reaction. Landon's little brother would just stare at the pandemonium, with a look of knowing something is just not right about this picture. During this period, we invited no one over except a spare few, nor did we leave the house unless necessary. (This never stopped people from stopping in!) We did this not only because we did not want anyone to endure the volume of his screams, but also because we did not want to scare anyone. Their fear would only add to ours and would be counterproductive to our goals. Eliminating the candida would not be an easy task and in retrospect I'm glad we started this sooner rather than later in the treatment.

After the second or third week of using the kefir, one day we noticed something peculiar. I sat down with Landon that night with a Scooby Doo book in hand. As we leafed through the pages, I pointed out the characters and said their names. "Shaggy", he said as I pointed to Shaggy. Ed looked up in disbelief as he picked up toys from across the room. Did he just say Shaggy? Our first breakthrough! He then started saying words here and there, and even started pointing to objects, something he never did before. Before this moment, he had been completely non-verbal, and would only repeat sounds. His mind appeared stuck in a loop. When he would try to speak, only words such as "ayyyyyyyyyyyy yayyyyy" or syllables put together would come out, never materializing into speech.

Our goal now was we needed to stabilize him at a low dose with minimal die-off and build up slowly until ultimately reaching the desired amount of four to six ounces a day. This seemed like an impossible task considering we could barely get through

½ teaspoon a day. I went back to that BabyCenter forum and kept reading what Kerri and others wrote about their experiences. It was identical to ours: crazy fits, yeast purging, then improvements in behavior. Each meltdown was followed by extreme improvements in mood. Like the other mothers' kids, Landon would also be happy even if it was just for an hour or two until the next episode. As difficult as it was, we knew inherently we had to push through this. When your wheels get stuck in the mud, what do you do? You stop, put it in reverse, back up, and start over slow. Repeating this in our heads became second nature.

I believe this is the most difficult yet most important part of our treatment program, and also where I think parents fall short. I could not help but think most parents must give up at this stage because they feel they are hurting their child. Years later I even spoke to a parent named Dave I met at the World Poker Finals who did just that. I happened to be seated next to him and noticed he had an autism awareness puzzle piece card marker. This prompted a discussion about autism, and we discovered we had something in common. We both had an autistic child we had on biomedical treatment. He described his son's reaction to the anti-fungal treatment as very similar to Landon's, as if he were being stabbed to death with a thousand knives. Going to the ER was not an option, for his fears of persecution were virtually identical to what we envisioned in our situation. What mainstream medical doctor is going to understand the unorthodox type treatment we have going on, and more importantly grasp the knowledge they mysteriously skipped over in medical school? It's ludicrous to even have to use the word "unorthodox" or "alternative" because it's so common sense to me, and this type of illogic made it more apparent that we live in a world where the truth often gets attacked, and at times transposed. Shouldn't using prescription drugs that don't heal you be called "alternative" treatment? Dave stopped antifungals and justified to himself that the diet was keeping his son calm, no more antifungal terror. I considered that a possible problem could lie here. Seeing the antifungals through to the end is where I believe the crossroads were, and could have made a recognizable difference. They stopped in fear of harming their son, as I chronicled earlier. I do not think he should have settled for "calm". In my opinion, you have to go through adversity to make gains. Dave told me the B12 injections (also a part of Landon's biomedical treatment plan) only seemed to make his son extremely hyperactive. This is a problem I remember reading about in our first stages with B12, that manifests if you do not clear up yeast issues beforehand. I never knew if this was true in our case because the die-offs were blamed first before anything else, for virtually every negative reaction we saw. Dave went through years of stress as well as thousands upon thousands of dollars worth of biomedical treatment for his son, only to stop with minimal benefit.

My question to them would be, would your son have recovered completely had you stuck with the antifungals? Was this the missing link that may have made the difference? He did not entertain this notion as seriously as I had hoped, as I threw more hints at him to maybe reconsider trying again. Instinct told me to grab him by the collar and shake him, urge him to go back and see it through. As a man with the knowledge he had, I did not feel it was my place to try and persuade him. His son was years older now, and I really did not know how effective treatment would be at this time. The question remained in my mind, if Dave read that BabyCenter forum like I did, would he have pushed through it?

Appearing defeated, he explained that during their treatment, their son's new doctor had informed him that he discovered something vital to his son's condition. Like a sad movie, they were supposed to meet about and discuss this at his office, however the doctor died suddenly before the appointment. I could not help but feel grief from his story. All I could say was, "I'm sorry", knowing words would be ineffective. Speaking with Dave about various biomedical terms was like speaking a foreign language at the card table. I suddenly noticed everyone was listening to us in silence trying to comprehend what we were talking about. We may as well have been speaking an African Bush language. Although there was a great difference in our dedication to the cause, it was refreshing to finally meet someone in my circle who shared the same knowledge I did. In fact, one important sentiment I continually felt throughout this whole process was an eagerness to share information. In my eyes, to withhold information or new insight from another parent was petty and grossly irresponsible. I used to work with people who held back from teaching others the ropes, always thinking this would get them ahead in the workplace. Not only did it not get them ahead in the workplace, it never got them ahead in life.

The antifungal treatments were by far the most backbreaking part of our journey. Coconut kefir and the sun proved to be our most powerful candida fighters. The morning after a day at the beach caused the most significant amount of detox, which was especially visible in Landon's eyelids. One of the many things I read and remember the mothers talking about in the Baby Center forum was that not only is it difficult to kill the yeast, but also to ward it off due to the spores. Once you have a Candida infection, you are always susceptible to it. Most of their success was due to the long-term antifungal treatment with Diflucan or Nystatin, lasting for months at a time. Bock mentions this time period is applicable with chronic Candida overgrowth, with systemic symptoms.[20] It was only when parents stopped using the antifungals prematurely that the yeast returned, sometimes worse than it previously was. This was the biggest reason I felt we could not stop.

As I drove home from doing errands one Saturday morning, I crossed off my list something I've been meaning to do. I called Michael Larsen, the man I saw on the Fox News YouTube video who used coconut kefir to help heal his daughter. He believed in it so much he started his own coconut kefir company, which was the only number I had to get in touch with him. Fate was on my side that day because he answered the phone. Apparently I caught him at a rare time because they were never there on weekends and usually had a staff there during the week. We spoke at length on the phone as I hurled questions at him regarding reactions.

I'm not sure if I was looking for an excuse to stop the kefir or looking to him for reassurance and motivation to trek on. He described his daughter's die-offs and disclosed the unsavory details about the amount of biofilm that she excreted after each turbulent episode. (So that's what the white excrement is, biofilm!) I was elated to finally be talking to someone concerning this, not just reading about it. I was also relieved to know we weren't killing our kid. This torture we were going through wasn't for nothing, we were gaining ground. He asked what age Landon was (18 months), and expressed shock that we were on top of this problem so early on. His daughter was four when they started and he said by age six, she was healed. I told him of my fears, anguish, and the sheer torture of watching Landon suffer through this horror every day.

Talking with him was a great boost as he was very encouraging. Most importantly, he gave me a lot of hope. I would think back to our conversation a lot as each crisis presented itself. During Landon's manic episodes I remember head banging, revolting spit up, hyperactivity, foul breath, head sweating, belly bloating, swollen lymph nodes, hives, inconsolable meltdowns, and an unquestionable and unmistakable odor coming out of his pores. I will never forget that distinctive smell. I really never understood exactly what the smell was caused by (Candida die-off or toxins?), but whatever the stench was, resembled rotten chemicals.

When Landon spit up the white biofilm type substance the gentleman spoke to me about during his daughter's episodes, it was the worst smelling of all. I did not think it was mucous because it was extremely difficult to wash off. Water alone could not break it down, so whatever this excrement was coming out of him was noxious to say the least. We discovered activated charcoal, which became our best friend and would usually mitigate the episode within a half hour. One or two capsules in hemp milk would usually do the trick. In addition to reading about it, Dr. C had also told us about using this. The charcoal, we were told, binds to the toxins and carries them out of the body immediately. The only problem with charcoal is that it prevents nutrients from being absorbed, so you cannot give it to the child right before or after a meal. Since that interfered with every meal of the day, we abstained from charcoal unless we absolutely could not handle the crazed flip outs.

According to Dr. Josh Axe (draxe.com), "activated charcoal is a potent natural treatment used to trap toxins and chemicals in the body, allowing them to be flushed out so the body doesn't reabsorb them".[21] This works through the process of "adsorption, the chemical reaction where elements bind to a surface."[22] He explains, "The porous surface of activated charcoal has a negative electric charge that causes positive charged toxins and gas to bond with it."[23] He notes, "Activated charcoal is not charcoal used in your barbecue grill. Barbecue charcoal is loaded with toxins and chemicals and should never be consumed."[24] (I thought this was worth mentioning in case somebody takes a piece of charcoal from their grill for their child to consume before their next meal!) As far as the dreadful smell from Landon's pores goes, we could bathe him five times a day and that potent smell would never go away. It was constantly being released from his body.

Landon's die-offs, I believe, resembled a yeast infection of the blood. It was literally everywhere in his system. I believe it was much worse than any of those BabyCenter mothers had with their kids. Even while cleansing, he was unable to function normally at a mental or physical level, and still digressing rapidly. I urge anyone who reads this to look up Candida stages 1-5 and see just how life threatening it really is. Mitchell Medical Group, hubpages.com, and candidacleanser.com all have articles sharing information about the stages of Candida overgrowth. Stage 1 is comprised of colic, rage, UTI's, eczema, thrush, allergies, and gas. Stage 2 becomes more severe, like the inability to gain weight, arthritis, and migraines. Stage 3 creates neurological problems, memory loss, anxiety attacks, violence, IBS, thyroid issues. Stage 4 moves onto adrenal/endocrine problems, "systemic yeast" and can affect the organs. In stage 5, the organs fail and death may result.

I believe we stopped Landon's candida at or before stage 4. His adrenals were so challenged, he couldn't be at peace for even a half hour out of the day. He refused to even climb the stairs on his own and his anxiety level was a nine out of ten all the time. I mentioned earlier about confusion between herxheimer and allergic reactions. When these die-offs or herxheimer reactions occurred, Landon would have hives everywhere so a lot of the time it seemed as if it was an allergic reaction to something else he ingested. Die-off or an allergic reaction? This confused us most of all and is a running theme throughout this book. I had to convince Ed to push on because hives is a symptom of yeast die-off just like a lot of those BabyCenter forum mothers described. Each time we hit this roadblock, I would go keep going back to the forum and read. The forum served for reassurance purposes during this dark time period. (I ultimately credited this forum years later for single handedly rallying me through the yeast obstacle.) Ed thought it was possible Landon was intensely allergic to coconut from the kefir. I argued no, because it took days for his reactions to occur initially. The difference to me was all his die-offs seemed to happen after a build up occurred. An allergy would be immediate. It was during this time frame, we convinced Dr. C to let us try a prescription antifungal. We wanted to see if maybe this did the job without the unfavorable reactions. She prescribed Nystatin, an antifungal she explained that purges yeast from the digestive tract. I was not happy with Nystatin, because I felt Landon had yeast throughout his system, not just his digestive tract. From what I read from those moms, it is Diflucan that clears out the system. We tried the antifungal for several weeks but all it did was form a red mark around Landon's mouth, like a clown. We eventually reverted back to the natural antifungal, coconut kefir.

The same question always circled back. Do we discontinue or do we continue? Not only were we dealing with possible allergic reactions, we might also be dealing with intolerance. Initially, we ended up discontinuing most supplements we tried, because we did not introduce them properly. We failed to give them to him one at a time, never knowing what reaction stemmed from what supplement. Instead, we gave them all at once never allowing enough time between supplements. Additionally, since Landon was already crazy from the detox, gauging the supplements' effectiveness was impossible. This became a constant obstacle for any new supplements we introduced later, even after properly administering them at three day intervals.

The mothers on that BabyCenter forum became my main source of emotional support. Their hardships were our hardships.

They were inspirational and supportive even though their stories were years old, and I was reading from the outside. We never took our foot off the pedal even though these episodes continued for what seemed like an eternity. Mostly due to the coconut kefir, Landon's healing reactions/die-offs (or whatever it was we were witnessing), lasted a year and a half, averaging three times a day, sometimes at two hour intervals. It was absolute torture to watch, and the worst part was you could not run away. Nevertheless, each episode gained way for new milestones. Again, two steps forward, one step back. I envisioned a pot of gold at the end of this rainbow. I had faith the craziness would indeed end one day, but knew it would not be that easy.

After many months of buying the costly commercial kefir, we decided to make homemade coconut kefir for ourselves. Why not get healthy at the same time and see just what this stuff does for us? Most likely I had Candida because of all the antibiotics and oral steroids I've been administered the last decade for lung infections. Landon did not just pick it up out of thin air. I had noticed lately I was extremely swollen or bloated, especially around the facial area, never making a connection that this may be an internal health issue.

We went to Whole Foods and bought the young green coconuts (they were white husks actually), drilled holes to extract the water, then fermented the coconut water with water kefir grains we purchased from eBay. If we stored the grains correctly, we could use them over and over indefinitely. This required rinsing them with filtered water, feeding them regularly with palm or coconut sugar, and never using metal. From what we read, metal kills the kefir grains. The art of fermentation and double fermentation became an education for us. Initially, not only were we not able to produce the fizz associated with coconut kefir, but the grains were dissolving after each bottle. Regardless, we still drank the liquid and it had a cleansing effect for sure. We remained unsure if the fizz was an important element or not to the fermentation being a success seeing as that the grains were still eating the sugar. After several trial and error runs, we were able to produce the fizz by adjusting to a warmer temperature. Upon opening the secured bottle we found that somewhere in between the kefir hitting the ceiling and just hearing a loud "pop", is exactly where we wanted to be. If you want to know if you've made the perfect coconut kefir, it should taste like the smell of stinky socks. Like the store bought kefir, ours really smelled just like dirty socks and it meant we were on the right track. The puzzle was now complete.

DETOX ME

After four months of ingesting eight ounces of coconut kefir a day, I had what is best described as a near-death detox experience. Coconut kefir delivered me a knockout punch. It was the closest I have ever felt to death and if I could have reached the phone to call 911, I would have. The morning started out fine, having showered, changed, and ready to take my daughter to her orthodontist appointment. As I gulped down my glass of kefir and a little kombucha, something happened. Instantaneously I felt a change come over me. Within seconds of downing the drink, my blood pressure and body temperature rapidly dropped off. An uncontrollable wave of fever/chills/shaking took over my body as I sat at the kitchen table shivering. This happened so suddenly and so severely I knew it could only be one thing... detox.

I had been waiting for this day to arrive, as the sentence "you are going to be sick" played back in my head from a gripping article I read about kefir. This was way beyond sick; this was what I thought would be my demise. The past several weeks I did notice I was making several more trips to the bathroom during the day. This was unusual for me, and in my opinion, was a foreshadowing of what was to come. I also remember reading the more toxic you are, the worse the Herxheimer effect will be. The illness came over me like a tidal wave, basically leaving me with no time to react. I had to leave in five minutes for that orthodontist appointment and was uncertain about my condition.

I decided to make the drive, despite the shivering and shakes that now commanded my body. My daughter showed no sympathy, asking me what was wrong and telling me to please try to get a hold of myself. Pre-teens are more embarrassed by their parents at that age than any other, so I'm sure she was just thrilled walking in with a mother who must have looked like a recovering drug addict. During this ride, I turned the temperature dial as high as it could go. I could not stay warm in 70 degree heat as my teeth chattered away. I made the drive safely, somehow averting disaster. Had I been pulled over, I am sure I would have been asked to exit the vehicle with my arms in the air while they tested me for driving under the influence. Honestly, it would have been safer driving under the influence than the condition I was in. As I sat in the waiting room, the noticeable stares I was getting from the staff were of no importance to me at that moment. I just wanted to get through that moment, as survival became my main focus. Unable to function or sit still, I told the assistant we had to go. I remember wondering if I resembled what a heroin addict looks like going through a withdrawal or detox, and if those receptionists were thinking the same. Although that did cross my mind, I did not care anymore. The challenge would be making it to the car and driving us home safely. Hallelujah, we did make it home.

As I walked inside, I told Ed I was really sick. His dismal reaction told me this would be my problem. Ed was busy that day caring for Landon and preparing his meals, so I needed to follow the routine and take care of my youngest son, Cole. The challenges lately had been overwhelming and he made sure to let me know I was not getting any pity from him. Lately, Ed and I were in each other's cross hairs, angry with one other and the world for what was happening in our lives. Whether he did not believe I was as sick as I was, or did not care, it was obvious I would have to figure out a way to look after Cole and at the same time take care of myself in my deathbed.

As it turned out, I was completely helpless and unable to take care of my youngest, who spent the day crawling around my room with the door shut. I struggled to stay warm as I stood in the piping hot shower for 45 minutes, still freezing cold. My head had fireworks going off inside and felt as if it were going to explode. My skin had been unbearably itchy all week in certain spots, and now itching so badly that lesions formed, expelling liquid, which I later determined was most likely yeast. This was eerily similar to what I noticed with Landon in those first few months and during his die-offs. The lesions had actually started weeks before, another precursor leading up to this fateful day.

This was the detox I was expecting, though I did not anticipate the force at which it would happen, nor the short amount of time it took to occur that morning. After four months, one would think I was in the clear. But it was this day my body cleansed itself through my skin, bowels, urine and vomit. My overloaded liver was finally unable to handle the surge of toxins dying off which I assume accelerated at too fast of a rate for my body to expel in a normal fashion. It was all coming out whether I liked it or not. At the end of this torment (one day), my liver discharged what I can only describe as a surge of hot acid along with acute stabbing pains for hours afterward. Without going into further details, my body purged out in one day what I had been building up for 40+ years. My mother happened to stop by later and had a look of alarm on her face when she saw me on the couch. "You don't look good at all." She actually checked up on me the next day to see if I was still alive.

The following morning I woke up feeling superhuman. If you put a cape on me, I could have leaped out the door and soared away into the blue sky. At least five pounds of garbage must have drained out of me. Ed stared at me in astonishment as if I had secretly performed some kind of overnight liposuction. I no longer had the inflammation around my face, and the weeping lesions were all gone. Little sparks were still going off in my head but only remnants of the fireworks the day before. I felt a level of purpose this day, a sort of connection, because I had walked in Landon's shoes. I could not believe that this little boy was going through nearly every day, what I had experienced just once. This gave me a newfound association and empathy for him. We were bonded.

I might add that during this time I was ingesting all this kefir, my youngest son's allergies completely went away while breast-feeding. Although his allergies were to a much lesser degree than Landon's (mostly characterized by large red spots on his face after eating), he did have them in the beginning. My conclusion from this was that I must have had some messed up gut flora and been very toxic when I had both of these kids. The only difference was I did not take any antibiotics or Prednisone while pregnant with my youngest.

Before my day of what I consider to be a detox, I suffered from depression. I was gloomy on a day to day basis never really having a reason behind it. From this day on, I became a different person, experiencing no feelings of depression since. My mind is no longer clouded as I notice how much more clearly I can think and better I can write. I am also calmer, not as uptight as before. Somehow I believe this all had to be linked to my emotional health as well, like that gut/brain connection mentioned earlier. Granted, I do a lot more for my health since, like probiotics, and vitamin B complex, but this moment was instrumental to super-charging me forward. This marked the beginning of when I started to examine general health and supplements more closely, as well as trying to get family to listen. It also made me question why doctors told me years earlier I needed to have my gall bladder removed. Why was that the answer and not a liver/gall bladder flush? Maybe a cleanse or a detox such as this would have done the trick. One doctor I dated for years even told me the gall bladder had absolutely no function or purpose to be there. Interesting, because ever since the day I had it removed, I have had nothing but digestive problems. Storing and releasing bile necessary for digestion is not a function? Was I being lied to here, or did he really believe this? If this surgery really was an example of most doctors' thought processes, I believe we are in danger. Something needs to be done before my lungs are removed to cure my asthma! I knew my job now was to look out for my health as well as my family's health. Nobody else was going to.

That day left me to only imagine what Landon's body was going through on a daily basis. He was getting only a fraction of coconut kefir that I had been taking, and we were giving him the weaker store bought coconut water kefir made from cultures which were safer (due to the fact you know exactly what strains you are getting). We tried ordering the cultures from Body Ecology to ferment the coconut water ourselves but it always turned out flat. The grains, on the other hand, had many more strains of bacteria. However, since it was unknown about the exact ones we were getting, we did not give this to him. During these months of turmoil, we knew kefir alone would not heal this child. He needed more help, just like Dr. C suggested. However, since most of the supplements we introduced during this time were met with adverse reactions, we were stuck in neutral. The detox alone was taking such a toll on his body, how could he regenerate and heal with a broken immune system being so sick all the time?

6

DIET

The next part of the treatment that was the easiest for us, but a nightmare for most, also happens to be the most important. I am talking about diet. Since Landon could barely eat any foods as it was without getting hives or feeling pain, we realized he was already by default eating what the GAPS diet calls for. Dr. Natasha Campbell-McBride's book "Gut and Psychology Syndrome" citing the "Specific Carbohydrate Diet"[25] developed back in the 1920's by Dr. Sidney Valentine Haas, explains how the diet can heal and repair leaky gut. We would follow this diet to a "T", because Landon's gut wouldn't allow for anything else. I would hear countless stories about parents who found this change in diet too difficult to institute and would discontinue the program. Trying to change a child's diet after they have been conditioned to eating a diet not in accordance with this program must be painstaking. I read stories about parents chasing their kids around the house trying to get them to eat a spoonful of green vegetables. Most of these kids were addicted to foods such as macaroni and cheese and fried foods. Bock explains the theory that the partial proteins in casein and gluten would intoxicate them because of their inability to fully digest them. Therefore, removing all casein and gluten from the diet of an autistic child is non-negotiable. Also important is that both parents need to be on the same page. One cannot be feeding the child vegetables and chicken while the other is serving french fries and soda. There is a very strict discipline involved in this process and any point you give in could mean a delay in healing the gut.

This diet was all Landon ever knew, so at least we caught a break in this regard. The GAPS diet has a list of foods which will not wreak havoc on the digestive system while your body works to repair the damage to the gut lining. Making adjustments to his diet like eliminating sugar and reactive foods, kept his eczema at bay. One wrong food and the rashes and scratching would return. Our plan was to keep him on this diet while cleaning him out, hopefully reversing the damage to his gut so he could eat and function normally. The foods Landon would eat were broccoli, cauliflower, turkey, and raw sauerkraut. Limited fruits with natural sugars (he needed some sugar) were fine which we gave sparingly, such as berries and apples. Natural limited sugars were acceptable as long as they were not processed. I believe eliminating processed sugar was the most important step in our diet plan for Landon. After removing it from my own diet, complications I suffered from drastically improved, and left me with a better overall feeling.

We were told Landon needed more protein, so the doctor recommended pea protein powder. This seemed to cause some pain and agitation when we introduced it into his food, so we had to stop. I tried introducing bone broth, which is extremely healing to the digestive system. I mentioned earlier that I first learned about bone soup listening to Ben's radio podcast. His description matched everything I read about online, a real healing super food. In my opinion it is quite possibly the world's perfect food. The benefits derived from it specifically aid the digestive tract. At first we ordered organic bone broth online from a place called Bare Bones, but later on in the program, I decided I would rather make my own. The process I decided on was to boil an organic chicken overnight for at least 12-24 hours and remove the chicken several hours into the process. Landon needed everything this soup had to offer like collagen, connective tissue, and the essential amino acids glutamine and cysteine. I remember Ben mentioning the last two specifically. Glutamine helps to seal the gut while cysteine is a powerful detoxifier.

However, like the coconut kefir, Landon's reaction to this was immediate and severe leaving us to question whether he was allergic to the chicken or whether it was a strong healing response. He would drop to the floor and had those all too familiar manic episodes, drenched in sweat and eczema flaring. We were not sure what to attribute this to since he was hyper-reactive to almost everything throughout the day. After that first bowl of broth it was back to square one. Maybe we were throwing too much at him at once. We backed off this one for now and reintroduced it later when he could tolerate more foods. My goal was to give this to Landon every day as there were too many benefits to this soup for us to abandon it altogether. Eventually that is just what I did and continue to do so to this day.

At age two, foods we knew he could not eat were…everything! We had been feeding him eggplant and squash for a long time before reading about GAPS. We later learned eggplant is what is referred to as a nightshade vegetable and should be avoided by people who have allergies or food sensitivities. Eggplants and bananas would create dark circles under his eyes, so we had to eliminate them both. Butternut squash was listed as a food to avoid as well, so we switched over to spaghetti squash. Rutabaga was an excellent anti-candida food for our son, but it was so labor intensive to peel, cut, boil and mash them three times a week that we decided to switch off for awhile. We did some reading on raw sauerkraut and discovered this is a high potency probiotic food. We started off at very small amounts, and were again confronted with the same demonic reaction. Was this a die off or an intolerance? This question again popped up and we were confronted with the decision to back off completely or reduce the amount. We knew this was good for him, so we reduced it to very little but still enough to get down. When it came to eliminating reactive foods, I am slightly opposed to Ben. Yes, I do disagree with him periodically! With people having general digestive issues, Ben's advice would be to target then eliminate the offending food. My objective takes it a step further. Instead of permanently eliminating the offending foods, why not heal the gut in order to make it possible to eat the foods not tolerable before? So in a perfect world, removing an intolerant food would only be temporary. Maybe I misunderstood him but I never heard him speak about bringing the reactive food back into the diet at a later time.

Ben mentions fermented foods at least once every show. I distinctly remember him saying they not only serve a probiotic value, but the food becomes more readily absorbed. I spotted an article called "Kefir, Kombucha and Sauerkraut: Fermented Foods for Your Heart Health"[26] by Ornish Living on huffpost.com. It explains the health benefits of the fermentation process of foods and beverages. Fermentation "enhances the food's nutritional value". In addition, the article explains that Omega-3 fatty acids, as well as key enzymes and B vitamins, are created in the fermentation process as well. We tried to make our own sauerkraut with cabbage and salt, which is really all that is needed. We stopped after our first batch because we basically did not trust our competency in this area. I was not at ease wondering if we screwed up the fermentation, which could result in bad strains of bacteria or spoiled sauerkraut. One important note about sauerkraut I remember hearing is to make sure it is the raw kind, only found in the refrigerated section of the grocery store, and not the kind you see on the shelves that are vinegar based. Miso soup was also included in our list of foods we successfully tried, something that Landon has always loved.

One discrepancy I found along this path was between Ben and Dr. Bock. While Ben was positively in favor of fermented vegetables, Dr. Bock did not include this in the list of diet related foods. I'm not quite sure of the reason behind this, especially considering the man in the YouTube video who healed his daughter with Dr. Bock's treatment plan, used fermented coconut water as part of the program. Since reading many positive articles about raw sauerkraut being a potent probiotic food, I decided using wild fermented foods would be beneficial going forward.

A very good healthy-fat food we gave Landon was avocados. The only bad thing about avocados is they turn brown fast so you really cannot store them in the fridge once you mash or cut them up. We tried blending it with banana and storing it in those small baby bullet containers. Eventually we decided it was easier not to store them at all. We would have to cut them up fresh every meal.

Coconut oil, also mentioned by Ben a lot, was the common denominator of every meal we served Landon. Whether it was cooking his food in coconut oil or feeding it to him straight, the benefits of this food are invaluable. Since I was now obsessed with yeast annihilation, I tried to incorporate anything coconut into his meals. According to candidadiet.com, coconut oil is one of the main yeast inhibitors/killers made by nature, containing three medium-chain fatty acids (Lauric, caprylic, and capric acid). These can be bought in supplement form as well. I prefer ingesting the oil the way nature intended. If Ed and I had to do this all over again, we would have blended together some coconut milk, coconut oil, kefir, turkey, and avocado and that would have been his formula as a baby. Later on, we would have added bone broth. In my opinion it would have been a much safer and healthier alternative than commercial baby formula.

We stopped the sugar formula when we learned just how much sugar was in it. He had been on special kinds prescribed first by his dermatologist, then by a naturopath doctor (one of a few in between I did not mention). What these doctors did not know was the sugar was promoting further destruction. How did a naturopath not know about this? If you look on the back of the label of any baby formula, it is loaded with sugar. What have we learned so far? Sugar feeds yeast which causes a mess of problems for the gut.

NATURAL CHELATION

Since Landon's labs indicated he had several heavy metals in his body, I wanted to at least try a natural form of chelation. Articles on naturalsociety.com, and from Natural Integrated Health Associates, discuss how cilantro coupled with chlorella, is a natural, cheap, and effective way to pull out heavy metals and stop them from reabsorbing. I read in these articles that both used together were very successful chelating agents and even had a more desirable result than if you were to use chelation IV. I tried green juicing with cilantro, kale, and fermented red cabbage juice for a few weeks only to get the same frenzy fit reaction from

Landon. The rashes and the manic fits were enough to make me abort the mission. Like the bone broth, I planned on considering this green juice in the future.

7

B12 INJECTIONS

Part of our biomedical treatment for Landon required subcutaneous methylcobalamin injections, a form of B12. As scary as it was for me at the time to administer, ultimately this is what I believe saved his life. The word shot or injection pains me to hear or say. This was the part of the plan that frightened me the most. Is it just B12 inside these injections? Because his immune system was so weak, I had reservations about injecting him with anything. We agonized over this for days before finally deciding to do it. A doctor has to prescribe B12 shots that come from a compounding pharmacy. Before injecting Landon, I called the pharmacy based out of New Jersey and asked them if there were any fillers, preservatives, or heavy metals in these shots. The pharmacist on the phone told me yes, benzyl alcohol is used as a preservative. I was stunned. Why was I never informed of this, and why was I the one who had to ask? She told me the FDA requires this so there was not much they could do about it.

Our biomedical doctor had told us the shot was straight methylcobalamin, nothing else. We called her to notify her of this, and she defiantly insisted there was no preservative. Her attitude was less than desirable, but we really did not have a choice at this point, we had to put up with it. She must have called the pharmacy because after she hung up the phone, she called back a little while later explaining apologetically that she was never informed of this change, and the FDA had her hands tied. This was our defining moment.

I remember being paralyzed with fear before Ed had to give Landon that first methylcobalamin shot. I equated shots with negative things automatically, so even if it was straight B12, it was a lot for my mind to handle. We sat for days contemplating how to get around this, thinking that maybe we can give him oral drops instead. As it was explained to us, this would not work because he could not absorb B12 through digestion, and it was imperative for brain function and detox. She also confirmed what I had read about B12. His body was not detoxing properly and these shots would help his system detox and improve neurological functioning. I remember reading biomedical doctors' stories about B12 and the immediate effects it had on children who were considered brain damaged. Shockingly, they were never brain damaged; they were B12 deficient. After several injections over three weeks time their cognitive functioning returned to normal. This information, and belief in our doctor's abilities, was enough to push us forward. The day arrived to give him that first injection. We were instructed the injection had to be done at a 45 degree angle for proper absorption, never straight down. (there are YouTube instructional videos of how to do this) I remember

Landon's face turning white as a ghost, perhaps gray. What was done was done, and there was no going back. Since I could not get the "thimerosol" and "shots" correlation out of my head, I also could not rid myself of the thought that I could have damaged Landon for life. I do not consider benzyl alcohol a neurotoxin but to a child whose life hangs in the balance, it suddenly became just as dangerous in my mind. The pharmacist did a good job convincing me that such a small amount will not harm my child. With Landon however, there was no such thing as a small amount of anything. What made me more nervous was, were they concealing anything else from me about what else was in that shot? The benzyl alcohol was hidden from me, so what else are they not disclosing?

The next day he was over the edge, and we both realized this may have been a catastrophic mistake. I must have bawled for two days straight on the phone with my mom telling her I think I just sealed his fate. She comforted me by saying to have faith in the doctor's analysis, and that I did what I had to do. Well, the shot must have been detoxed him in some fashion because the following day he was like a different kid. He wasn't irritable, he wanted to play, he was walking straight, and was generally happier. We couldn't believe it. After cursing this doctor for a weekend, I had to apologize to her in my head and believe she knew what she was doing. I called her up that week to tell her about Landon's initial adverse reaction and she berated me for questioning her. She mentioned he was not supposed to have a bad reaction and suggested hydroxycobalamin as a substitute. This is just great. We finally get over the B12 hurdle and now she wants to give him a different form of B12 injection? I had not read up on that form and never heard Ben talk about it. After researching B12 to death before administering Landon the shot, the last thing I wanted do was give him a different injection.

Everywhere I read mentioned methylcobalamin as the purest and best form. I did not know enough about hydroxycobalamin to agree to do this.

We stuck to the methylcobalamin. Suprisingly, after each shot, Landon would be more irritable than content. He would have short spurts of happiness then miserable until the next shot (every three days). We tried stopping a few times to see what happened. After approximately a week he would start losing weight fast and regressing. I could not understand the B12/weight connection, nor could I understand how it seemed to create negative responses. These injections were supposed to be doing the opposite. I was told Landon is going to feel so much better, and should be "eager to hand deliver me the injection!" That should tell you how good the B12 should make him feel. How could something seem to help him and at the same time appear to be hurting him as well? Reading numerous articles I assumed we had to resolve the yeast issues first, otherwise it seems to exacerbate the tantrums and hyperactivity.

After a multitude of emails and calls to our doctor's office, I gave up trying to communicate. She was too abrasive for us to handle and not forthcoming about many topics, so I closed the chapter on her and reached out to Dr. Bock, the miracle doctor. I called his office the next day and made an appointment.

When I spoke to the secretary, she told me to make sure Landon fasts the morning we bring him in. Impossible, I thought, Landon will throw a tirade the entire car ride there without his bottle, and would never agree to drink only water. He maintained position in the driver's seat, even at age two, especially when it came to his bottle. After weighing the positives and negatives of our options, regarding the consequences of his behavior, we ultimately submitted.

I notified the receptionist we would bring him in for an office visit but no blood will be taken that day. The overnight fasting and long car ride would not be a good combination prior to a blood draw. Attempting it on a miserable child pushed to his brink could detonate a lethal outburst beyond anything imaginable. Plus, we tried countless times in the past and had little success. We could provide blood from the previous biomedical doctor, but knew we did not have enough for a thorough analysis. When I say thorough, I am talking not two or three vials of blood, but rather 12-14 vials. I remember the lab technician was shocked at the amount we had to draw, considering Landon's age. Even the lab technician was shocked at this. I guess biomedical doctors are used to this reaction, and maybe that's why Bock had his own lab and people to do the drawing. Holding Landon down would be hard enough, but to relive his screams would be too much to handle at the moment. (One time a phlebotomist kept missing the vein and had to poke him again and again!) Additionally, the blood will not flow when a body is under that much stress.

I'm still trying to figure out how these parents who take their kids for biomedical treatments are not only able to get the blood draw accomplished, but also able to get their kids on the airplane cross-country. Patients come from all over the world to see Dr. Bock so I'm assuming there has to be some level of sedation involved. I'm fairly certain Landon would have caused the plane to make an emergency landing. Once he goes over the edge, he cannot be calmed down to any extent.

On the day of our appointment in Red Hook, NY, we started the hour and a half drive early that morning. I will not lie; biomedical doctors can be costly and there's always the risk it will not work, but there was no price I would not pay to heal my child or at least try. For two or three weeks prior we had been giving him the coconut kefir probiotic as well as some supplements we had from the last doctor. He had been pretty close to impossible to tolerate and was himself in pain. Again, we never could tell whether it was a bad reaction to a certain supplement or if it was that darned never relenting die-off from the kefir. With so many variables, we were confused. Do we take him off everything and start over with Bock or do we continue with the kefir at least?

At Bock's office Landon was miserable. He was crying, whining, and had a constant need to be held. Nothing made him happy, and it became apparent we may not even make it through the appointment. It was a good thing for Dr. Bock to see, as I thought it would make his diagnosis and treatment easier, similar to when you take your car into a repair shop for a noise it's making, and when you get there it stops. We did not have to worry about this happening. However, with no blood work, he did not have much to go on. What I was able to hear above Landon's screams was a goal to heal Landon's gut, while in the meantime supplying him with the nutrients he is being deprived of. This was very similar to Dr. C but with different supplements.

Dr. Bock ordered new labs and $5k worth of blood work to be drawn. Be aware blood work can be very expensive when you decide to walk in the door of a biomedical doctor. The cost varies depending on what doctor you use but the one thing in common between all of them is that they all do a very detailed, comprehensive blood draw, as opposed to one from a regular practitioner (basics). The answers this extensive blood work offers are important and something to consider before you decide to walk away. The blood draw issue was my weak spot and something which I associated with defeat. I knew we just could not get past this. It would take three people to hold him down and the veins would be too difficult to find. With our last blood draw, the blood stopped flowing even when the nurse found the vein. Dr.

Bock also wanted us to schedule a separate appointment with the office nutritionist to go over Landon's diet. This was a separate fee and in my opinion an unnecessary expense. Diet should be incorporated as part of the initial visit and not a separate one. I was a bit taken aback by this considering he wrote all about specifications concerning diet in his book. You do not need a nutritionist to tell you about the GAPS diet or what Dr. Bock can lay out for you in five minutes. I did not like this at all, but hid my discontent.

After a few minutes of sulking and brooding about the necessity of the blood work, Dr. Bock asked us to tell our story. I told him what happened from beginning to end and how we arrived at where we were. He asked what I thought was the reason for Landon's problems. I told him when I was pregnant I was given antibiotics and prednisone and I was certain this was somehow the cause of his autism or autistic type behavior. He asked another question. Did I get a yeast infection? Yes I did! I paused for a few moments as I contemplated that question again. He did not have to say another word, I understood what happened. I understood what he was not telling me.

During pregnancy, I got a yeast infection from being treated with antibiotics (Augmentin) and Prednisone for a lung infection. I'm assuming Landon most likely did as well in utero. I treated my symptoms on the surface, (unbeknownst to me it was everywhere) but Landon was never treated. I cannot believe I never made that connection. I knew he was full of yeast from my intake of these substances but did not make the association to the infection I got. In the back of my mind I remember hearing about dangers of antibiotics to gut bacteria, but I never knew how dangerous. What had begun as useful information was now evolving into an education playing back in my head. From what we learned earlier, antibiotics destroy the gut flora which is the core of our immune system. Bock reiterates from an earlier chapter, "antibiotics kill not only disease-causing bacteria but also healthy bowel bacteria allowing yeast to take over."[27] Their message was the same. Everyone has good bacteria and bad bacteria in their intestinal tract. I devastated this balance between the two. I cannot say for sure this was the cause of all Landon's problems, but I was fairly certain it was the smoking gun. I will never know or pretend to understand the pain and suffering this child went through. Believing I caused this, I was determined to fix it.

8

REGRESSION

Dr. Bock asked questions, but he never communicated well with us. I felt as if I were pulling teeth trying to get answers out of him to explain why the supplements and medications he gave us were necessary, and what was their purpose? I made sure to research every supplement he gave us and what each one was responsible for because we were only given instructions on usage.

Calcium/Magnesium	Prim Royal
Probiotics	Pyridoxal 5 Phosphate
Ghee Butter	Megafolinic
Acid Reflux prescription	L-Methylfolate
Magnesium Taurate	Sonic cholesterol
Digestive Enzymes	

The first supplement he gave us was calcium/magnesium. I remember they are taken together for their symbolic action to aid the cardiovascular system, blood pressure, bone strength, nerve function, and building the immune system. Since Landon could not drink milk or obtain calcium from food, this was important.

Ghee butter was recommended for fats, but was vetoed within 2 days of trying. We were going to have to find a proper fat substitute for that later. Next on the list was a supplement called magnesium taurate, something I read is essential for brain growth and administering calming effects.

To our surprise he attributed Landon's back arching and pain to acid reflux. He prescribed an acid reflux medication to be taken daily before meals. Ed and I looked at each other in silence both knowing what the other was thinking. That prescription would never be filled. I precisely remember Ben saying never interfere with the body's natural ability to produce stomach acid, and that we need stomach acid to digest our food. Ben's ability to explain his rationale was exactly the reason why his ideology trumped everyone, including Dr. Bock. As it was, Landon was not digesting his food adequately, so this was a no-brainer. Had Bock communicated to us why this was the best option, we may have considered it. I even questioned if acid reflux had anything to do with Landon's intestinal pain. We kept this to ourselves knowing it was in our best interest to not question his expertise. We needed him and the last thing we wanted to do right now was put him off.

Finally, he told us to stop everything we had him on for a few weeks, including the kefir, before starting these supplements. This did not sit well with me because I felt in my soul that cleansing him was the single most important ingredient in his recovery. From everything I read, if I had to choose one thing to give him, it would be the coconut kefir. Even though the die-off seemed to make him crazy and impossible, he would dramatically improve afterwards. We also noticed the die-off episodes occurred less with more space in between them. Keeping him on the kefir would be our most difficult task but proved to be the most beneficial for his progress. I made the decision not to stop giving this to Landon for the long term, but agreed to stop it for a few weeks.

After stopping all supplements temporarily, his behavior was a total turnaround, and it was like having a normal kid in the house. He started counting and saying the alphabet and talking more. He wasn't healed, but it was a substantial difference to notice something changed. Ed's stance again, going back to chapter five, was that Landon had been allergic to coconut all along and that is why he couldn't tolerate the effects. He concluded this based on Landon's change in behavior from bad to good. I repeated my argument that this was unlikely because these reactions always start a few days after we give him the kefir, not immediately. We felt like broken records, continuously addressing the same concerns as if stuck in the same loop. From Dr. C to Dr. Bock, we kept running into the same brick wall. I felt it was important that I needed to repeat myself until Ed understood. I emphasized to him that as long as we continued giving him the kefir, the intolerant behavior would remain constant until the toxins were out and his blood was cleansed. Ben often brings up the term "congested blood" along with "cleansing the blood". I knew this had to be what was taking place. What I had thought all along was Herxheimer or die-off maybe was just a cleansing effect? Perhaps they were the same thing? The answer to this remains a mystery, something I never figured out. All I knew was what I am describing. Upping the dosage was increasing the calamity of his behavior so we had to make constant adjustments to the dosage to keep his die-off at a minimum. Insistent we had to keep going, I stuck to my guns. I would not abandon ship! Starting and stopping the treatment of cleansing him was making it worse each time we would start again. That only convinced me we had to stick to the course and double down on the dosage even if it meant having an impossible kid for a few months. The intensity of this die-off was like being caught in a blizzard. It was unbearable to endure, which is why we had to keep going. Had we not seen gains, then absolutely I would have said quit. But we were seeing progression, therefore we did not stop. We stuck to the kefir, and before long built the dosage up to six tablespoons a day.

Meanwhile, the blood draw for Bock's labs was a disaster. Listening to Landon's frenetic screams was as difficult as getting his veins to flow. After two attempts and three people holding him down, we gave up and decided just to proceed forward with the supplements regardless. The point of the blood draw was to narrow our focus. For now we would be at a slight disadvantage without this information.

INTESTINAL CLEANSE

Meanwhile, I heard another doctor on a podcast who developed an intestinal cleanse product called Oxy Powder. It's an oxygen based intestinal cleanser designed to clean out the years of undigested food lining in our guts. It's completely safe and non habit-forming, unlike laxatives. This doctor suggested an intestinal cleanse to anyone having health issues. Once you clean out your gut, your natural flora has a chance to flourish and do its job again. Back to the gut issue again. Now we have another doctor talking about the importance of gut health. I ordered this for Landon and for us to try. Once again Ed and I argued about giving this to him. Ed did not think it was necessary because he did not think Landon was constipated. I argued he needed a cleanse due to his bloated belly.

The oxygen is a natural candida killer as well and would be beneficial to use regularly. I went online and read about other parents who gave their children this supplement. I read nothing negative, only positive stories about how that was a very important supplement in their treatment program. Landon's diapers should have been sent to a forensic lab after taking this for a week. What comes out in the diaper and how it comes out should tell you everything you need to know about your child's health. I'm not sure what came out of Landon but Ed described the smell as that of a dead animal and taking on colors from dark green to black. The oxygen produced a die-off almost the same intensity as the kefir. Due to temporary insanity, we picked this point in time to wean him from the bottle of hemp milk he had hanging out of his mouth day to day. With the bottle he would drink non-stop, but transferring over to a cup brought the drinking to a complete halt. Since we mixed all his supplements into the hemp milk, the bottle would remain a necessity for the time being. We continued giving it to him for bedtime and morning, as it was the only way to get him to drink! Once we took it away, he would not voluntarily drink from a cup. We had to hold the cup up to his mouth and tell him to drink. He was sweating a lot, and the supplement would cause 3-5 bowel movements a day, so I know he needed liquids.

During one of our follow up phone conversations, Dr. Bock warned us to be prepared for "regression". Landon will appear to be going backwards at times even after improvements. I think this goes back to the two steps forward, one step backward proverb I mentioned earlier, but now it was more like one step forward, two steps backward. To a degree, we had already been living through regression with the kefir, but I'm glad he told us this. There were times we wanted so badly to quit, thinking the regression was permanent, or that we landed in a worse spot from where we started.

Here are examples of some things we experienced during regression. Landon would repeat the last word of a question I would ask him. If I asked him, "Landon do you want to go for a ride?" he would repeat the word "ride" back without understanding the question. Or, if I said, "do you want to go to the playground or the library?" he would mumble out a garbled word that sounded like library. Whatever the last word we would say happened to be, that would be the word he would repeat. Also, he would become fixated on something in particular (OCD), sending his world into chaos if we did not figure out what he wanted or what was missing. He would have a meltdown until we navigated back and made his world right again.

Incapable of handling his screams one day, we put Landon in his room and shut the door. Unable to get out, we heard loud bangs. We realized he was ramming his head into the door. This was not a child banging their head to get attention, Landon had no control of himself. The amount of blunt force he was using to try and move the door open was petrifying. What was even more chilling was that he was oblivious to the pain. Reading these stories from parents as opposed to actually living the horror really puts you in a different place. Seeing it happen changed me. Never quite sure what was lurking around the corner, times like these felt like a horror movie with no ending. The only thing I took comfort in was that this crazy behavior might cease if we stopped everything cold turkey. The fact was, more questions remained than answers. Would stopping everything stunt his overall progression? Was this all part of the regression Bock told us about, or were they new problems not associated with regression? Were we now going to have to start protecting Landon from himself?

In addition to the head banging, I noticed he would walk on his toes like a lot of autistic kids do, but it would only last a fleeting moment. This only happened a few times and then stopped. I also noticed the strange way Landon's eyes moved. When he spun in circles, his eyes would look out the corners in the opposite direction of which way he was spinning. He would often look up towards the ceiling so all that was visible were the whites of his eyes. I remember reading in Dr. Bock's book that this was a vitamin A deficiency. According to Bock, Vitamin A supplementation heals the function of the cones and rods in the eyes, which are commonly damaged in autistic children.[28] I also remember reading from the moms in the Baby Center forum this may be a yeast issue. A lot of things we saw in conjunction to Landon's regression included behaviors I just do not know how to articulate. Occurring routinely were instances of Landon simultaneously shaking his head and hands, as he raised them in the air, while making incoherent noises. Hyperactive spurts of running around the bedroom late at night in repeated patterns, was another problem we faced associated with die-off and this unrelenting backslide.

CARRY ME

Our most challenging task during this phase was Landon's persistent need to be carried around and held. Behaviors he adopted such as this could be categorized as OCD. Starting as a baby and continuing until age three, Ed and I were opposed when it came to this matter. I felt it was a control issue on Landon's part, whereas Ed knew holding him was consequential to his healing. Because of that belief, he became the Landon's master caretaker. Little did Ed know, he just waived his rights as a free man. The attachment phase had been activated, and like crazy glue, Landon became completely fastened to only Ed from this point on. Ed was sentenced to the next two years of no freedom, no chance of parole, and all time to be served under Landon. Going forward, Landon rarely allowed anyone else but Ed to carry him or care for him in general. We could never adjust our roles or alternate kids, almost similar to a hostage situation for Ed. It was easier that I took care of our younger child Cole, and Ed be the one with Landon most during this difficult period of time. Landon grew so accustomed to Ed, he would not allow him to eat, breathe, or use the bathroom without being held. If those needs were not met, there would be hell to pay. That extended to never allowing Ed to leave the house, go to the store, or put him down for two seconds without melting down. The store is another story within itself. You want to talk about making it to kindergarten? How about making it through a grocery line during this journey?

As I was preparing lunch one afternoon, I heard the door open and slam as Ed came inside. A look of horror was on his face. Another trip to Whole Foods was a nightmare. He spoke out to me, "you should see the look on the faces of the people at the register. I know they see me coming, they are praying I won't come through their line. Landon's screams can be heard miles away. He is out of his mind". I could see Ed's eyes welling up as he described the incident. This really hit home for him. When Landon was a baby, I had it happen to me too, in the grocery line. An elderly woman behind me clamored, "Please stop that baby from crying!" as she held her ears. It's interesting we had these experiences because I rarely recall seeing a parent with an autistic child running errands or going to the store. I wonder if this is why? I do know the post-traumatic stress from days like this still haunt us. Ed has blocked it all out now, which is why we are not co-authoring this book. His shoulder still bothers him to this day from carrying Landon and I'm not sure if he remembers why! I might add we were both lucky to not have to work due to fortuitous circumstances in my life. I'm not sure how we would have dealt with this situation had we both been working a 9-5 job.

By this time, the weeping lesions on Landon's face were a distant memory, but the die-off or cleansing caused the eczema in other places to get worse at times. I mentioned earlier in the book, we would have to put hair ties around his ankles to keep him from scratching, and put long socks on his hand and arms at night. If we failed to do this, he would mutilate himself by morning. Interesting to note, we had originally used those socks and ties when the yeast infection was building, now Landon had to endure it again as it was all releasing. It was clear everything bad had to reverse itself out of his body.

Most of the supplements Dr. Bock gave us never made it far. We were not sure if it was the brand of product we used, or if Landon was reacting to something else, or it was a continual healing crisis and he was perfectly fine with all the supplements. This time, we allowed the three days between each new supplement, however the detox turmoil going on inside of Landon still would not relent. The same dilemma of not being able to figure out cause and effect from any one supplement, made the implementation process infeasible. For a second time, we hastily abandoned all of the supplements because Landon was in a constant reactive state. We felt defeated. How in the world do any parents who choose the biomedical route continue this impossible uphill battle? In hindsight, I'm sure it was mostly due to the healing crisis and probably not the supplements or the brands.

Some of them, like digestive enzymes, could have been utilized had we stuck with it. I tried these for myself and was doubled over in stomach pain after multiple trials. Never knowing why or if Landon was affected the same way, I stopped the enzymes for both of us. (Later, when Landon was doing much better, we were able to successfully reintroduce the supplements with a different doctor and positive results. We followed the guidelines of leaving a three day gap in between each supplement so as to make sure we knew exactly what Landon could tolerate.)

I can see how many parents might give up at this point. We were constantly throwing our hands up in the air in frustration and wondering if anything at all is really working. We had so many questions for Dr. Bock which we were asked to email but took 1-3 days to get an answer. I believe the delay in his responses had a lot to do with having so many clients. He works with adult patients as well as children, so it likely made it impossible for him to cater to each and every individual. Lost in the shuffle, we decided to move on from Dr. Bock. Sadly, I'm not sure he realized we even dropped out. This never stopped me from referring him or pointing other parents in his direction. It would give me an excuse to hand out his book and really get parents to listen.

THE BEST LIE EVER

The day I met Maren was the turning point in my life. While rollerblading down a path in my town, I skated past a woman pushing a boy in a jogging stroller. He was feeble and sick looking, staring into space. Normally, I would mind my own business, but this time, something inside told to me to stop and get involved. I hesitated but continued on my way. Later that night, I ruminated over the way the child looked, thinking he might have the wrong doctor and the wrong course of action. Mad at myself for not stopping, I knew I must try and communicate the information I held. If I had to force myself to talk to people, so be it. As bad as my communication skills were, especially in face to face social interaction, helping people would start here for me. Because he was so young, surely the right doctor could help him. Next time, if I was allowed a next time, I decided I would say something.

As luck would have it, the following day I saw them again on the same path. This time I stopped. I needed to get the woman to listen. To do this, I had to approach this on a personal level she could relate to. "Does he have allergies?" I asked. I assumed he had gut issues based on his condition, so allergies had to be a definite yes. She seemed surprised and told me he did. I replied "my son does too and was just like him (pointing to the child) before we found the right doctor in NY and got him the proper help." I waited for her to digest my words as I knelt down to say hi to the boy. "What's his name?" The lady, who was his caretaker, said his name was Maren and he was five. I noticed Maren smiling at me, but his eyes were unable to meet mine as they looked off in different directions. He could not speak and obviously could not walk, he was a skeleton figure. I noticed he repeatedly scratched between his knuckles, something I vaguely recall reading about in relation to yeast. My immediate instinct told me it was autism. After talking for a few minutes about allergies, I went on my way. Hopefully she would relay my message back to his mother and she would be inquisitive enough to take action.

The following day as I drove my car up to the path, I saw the caretaker sitting on the bench and Maren next to her in his stroller. She had a pen and notebook in hand. It worked! She had indeed told the mother. Immediately, her questions began. "What is the name of the doctor I spoke about?" "Where is he located?" "Can my son walk now?" I gave her all of Dr. Bock's information including the type of doctor he was, his phone number and that he could be found in Red Hook NY. I learned during our conversation that day, Maren had a disease or condition I had never heard of. I sat back in shock that what I thought resembled low-functioning autism was something else. Flashback to earlier when I mentioned people who are told about rare conditions they have, like the "Bellibloatitis Inflamarxinomous" mock reference. What if the doctors felt forced to assign a label on something unknown to them? What if this was a complete autoimmune breakdown? Aware I was sounding more and more like Ben (a good thing!), I realized my rationale had changed and I was looking at everything from a brand new point of view. Picture a freshly picked growing apple in front of you. No longer getting nutrients from the tree, the soil, and the sun, it begins to rot or break down. You can give the condition of the apple names as it rots, like "Fruit Fascilitis" or "Turnbrown" syndrome. But the reality is, the apple is breaking down with nothing to sustain it. How is that different from us? I knew in my heart that whether Maren had this syndrome assigned to him, or it was something else completely, Dr. Bock could help him. This boy's body was starving of nutrients, and they were obviously on the wrong path. I know it was completely wrong to lie about Landon's condition being similar to Maren's, but it was a virtuous lie. I did what I had to do, and in my opinion the only way necessary to get them help. I did not enjoy lying in a dire situation like this, but if it put them on a path to healing, it was a necessary evil. At the very least, they were headed in the right direction.

I never saw them again after that. After moving away and returning years later, I looked, but they disappeared without a trace. I'm hoping and praying they went to see Bock. Even though he did not work out for us, I knew they were in good hands. He was one of the reasons we found the right path, and his approach is what the title of his book describes, groundbreaking.

9

HOLISTIC TRY

I n the interim of biomedical doctors, when Landon's progress hit a plateau, we decided to try a more holistic approach. I searched for doctors in CT who practiced holistic medicine, and found one who was an MD as well in Woodstock, CT. He was a licensed physician, surgeon, and homeopathic physician I will call Dr. S. We felt better going into this knowing he was an MD who understood biology and this was not going to be some pseudo witch doctor. His role or purpose to us mainly at this time between biomedical doctors was to decipher the blood work we were able to draw from Dr. C. Speaking with her was a lost cause and probably would have cost us another $1k just to go over the results. The costs incurred from her appointments made us feel as if treating our child was secondary to running a business. All the appointments seemed to last one to two hours and her charges per hour were excessive. Since we were never able to draw blood for Dr. Bock, we took what we had to Dr. S.

Dr. S's visit, to say the least, was disappointing. I remember his office was more like a house in the middle of nowhere. To his credit, he was the one who first mentioned the possibility of Landon having what is called an MTHFR mutation. I recall reading about this from a mother on that BabyCenter forum I would often refer back to, but I never bothered to research it. He suggested we might want to test Landon for this defect because he would need a specific treatment if he did test positive. Obviously, he saw signs in Landon that pointed to that mutation defect.

Later, I went home and read up more on this from a credible site I trust. On globalhealingcenter.com, Dr. Group explains, "if you have an MTHFR gene mutation, an inability to process folic acid (vitamin B9) can have serious consequences. A deficiency in B9 can cause a growing fetus to develop neural tube defects. The MTHFR gene is responsible for converting vitamin B9 (folic acid) into a form your cells can use for metabolism."[29] I already knew Landon's metabolism was screwed up. I had no doubt this may be playing a role in what was wrong here. I continued to read on about this on his site and learned folic acid combined with B12 is crucial for methylation in people with this defect. Dr. Bock really nailed down how important this function is in his book. I recall him saying that once methylation is repaired it can rescue countless children from severe problems. Considering a lot of autistic kids have this defect, think about how many uninformed parents could benefit from knowing this! I remember him talking about glutathione, along with methylation and its role in detoxing the body of toxins and heavy metals. I'm sure the 1 methylfolate he gave us had something to do with the B12 injections Landon was supposed to be receiving. We had stopped the injections along with almost everything else at that point because Landon was such a mess. A pattern started developing now between doctors. Obviously Landon needed B12 and folic acid. All three doctors so far had mentioned this as part of their approach. Dr. S explained there was a DNA testing site we could order from called 23andme. It would involve a pinprick of blood, but it's a relatively easy test, and we would know for sure if Landon did have this mutation.

After showing him the blood work, and explaining Landon's situation again, (with each doctor's visit, details were starting to get lost in translation) his matter-of-fact response was as follows, "Landon needs a fecal transplant". With most typical parents, this comment would have induced some sort of horrific reaction to the word transplant alone, but little did he know I was well read up on this subject. Unfortunately, this procedure is rare in the United States. Only a very small percentage would qualify and Landon would not fall under the qualifications. I do think he would have benefited greatly from this procedure to re-colonize his gut, however you cannot just walk into a doctor's office or medical facility and ask for a fecal transplant for your child. "Fecal transplantation", as JohnsHopkinsMedicine.org explains, "is the transfer of stool from a healthy donor into the gastrointestinal tract for the purpose of treating recurrent C. difficile colitis. When antibiotics kill off too many good bacteria in the digestive tract, fecal transplants can help replenish bacterial balance".[30]

First of all, C difficile was not present in Landon's stool so he would not qualify on that issue alone. Secondly, I'm not sure of the dangers regarding donors, or allergies to the donor's diet, or medical history of the donor. Because of the high success rate, this was something I considered but had to rule it out. I looked back at the doctor in amazement. The scare word "transplant" did nothing to faze me and I asked him, "In all seriousness, how would you expect us to find a doctor who would agree to perform this procedure without any of the qualifications? You need to be on a list and even then it's not a sure thing." Also, the FDA is also driving a wedge into the mix with regulations. This statement served no purpose other than to scare or demoralize us.

He really had no answers, which infuriated me. When you throw out a suggestion of that magnitude, you should be prepared to follow it. Put some action into your words! Had he offered to perform the procedure I would have taken him up on it, no questions asked. Instead, we left his office with something called lycopodium as well as instructions to order a certain brand of liquid methylfolate. We gave it a try but never seemed to make any headway. The drops needed to be diluted and I remember wondering how much water are we diluting the drops in, and how in the world was this supposed to work? As far as lycopodium goes, I'm not quite sure what it was or what it did but we never used it. Neither of us understood the healing significance of this herb.

My thoughts about lycopodium or any herbal medicine is as follows: When your body is deficient in essential vitamins and minerals you are comprised of, there certainly isn't anything an herb can do to heal or cure your condition. Our visit that day was a contributing factor in this conclusion we drew. I knew Landon had a biochemical problem and no herb or drug will fix that. He needed nourishment and a functioning metabolism. We needed answers, and we needed to see progress. It was maybe one more phone call with Dr. S before I told him we would be moving on. His last words to me were "Landon is a very sick child.", as if this was going to influence our decision to leave. Yes, I understood this, but he really did not give us a treatment plan. Mostly, I felt this would move very slow and time was of the essence. Dr. S definitely knew his stuff, but he failed to provide any type of specific guidance. At the time we were looking for aggressive treatment, and he was way too passive. We needed someone who dealt with this on a daily basis, and had the confidence to tell us what is going on, what we need to do, and be our cheerleader every step of the way.

Although at times it felt like we were running in place, not all was lost in these visits to multiple doctors. Each one was able to offer something valuable for us to hold onto and utilize. The common denominator every doctor emphasized was the gut-brain connection. An article from Anthony L. Komaroff (Editor in Chief of Harvard Health Letter, the Harvard Health Publication, Harvard Medical School) talks about this gut brain connection and that "A person's intestinal distress can be the cause or the product of anxiety, stress, or depression. A troubled intestine can send signals to the brain, just as a troubled brain can send signals to the gut. That's because the brain and the GI system are intimately connected."[31]

There does seem to be communication going on between the two for sure. Why is repairing his gut so difficult to do? This healing was going to take years, not a quick overnight fix. We stored away most of these supplements because at some point we figured they may come back into play. We kept them in the house as a reminder to order them again after expiration. A lot of these doctors prescribed the same ones, just different name brands. Those were the supplements we kept and continued to try, like digestive enzymes, probiotics, vitamin A, and vitamin C. Dr. Bock inadvertently introduced us to coconut kefir from his Fox News YouTube video, yet never approached us with this subject in his office. I'm sure that's because it inexplicably comes later in the treatment, but we bailed on him too early to find out. B vitamins were also prevalent in all these doctors' plans for Landon, so we incorporated these as best we could. Each new supplement carried its own allure that maybe this is the game changer, mak-

ing us over zealous to try them all out at once. As mentioned earlier, that was a mistake. One at a time, and you will do fine. The
bad news is that nothing happened overnight. This held true until we met our next doctor who was on the ball, and able to
uncover a major oversight. Even with that said, many things had
to come together over a period of time.

10

IT'S IN THE STARS

Landon's early years tested us in every way. The emotional ups and downs cannot be described by words. One day your child is lost in his own little world of repetition and fog, and the next minute the clouds lift for a moment as you see gains, and hope returns. Then it's back to gloom and doom, and whatever fleeting moments of elation you felt are gone, as regression rears its ugly head again. This new school of hands-on education was teaching me something. This was all part of the healing process, and behavior came first.

Most of Landon's gains came in his third year after we moved to Florida and found our new doctor, a true pioneer in his field. After six months of fighting my ex husband Tom (now one of my biggest supporters for Landon) in court for the right to move our daughter Angela out of state, we all packed up and moved to a place called Crystal Beach, a small community within the larger area of Pinellas County. We found a nice home on the inlet of the Gulf of Mexico right across the street from the water. The main reason for moving was to introduce Landon to nicer weather, closer to the ocean and the saltwater. We thought maybe this could prove beneficial to his overall health and we could clamp down on our treatment plan.

The road trip there was a blur. Driving from Connecticut to Florida through the night with deranged tantrums going on in the backseat was something we both blocked from our memory. We know we made the drive but are not sure how we got there. I remember it being very dangerous because we drove straight through, functioning on very little sleep. There was no other alternative due to the unrelenting die off episodes we still experienced from Landon. I believe this car ride may have been the most trying 24 hours of our lives as this appeared to be near the peak of Landon's healing crisis. What caused the man-on-fire screams to take place every few hours, I don't know. We accepted the possibility this would be a never-ending part of the treatment we would have to endure for the rest of our lives. I even bargained with God saying I would be fine with Landon never being able to talk as long as his suffering stops.

The last 45 minutes before arriving at our destination was like completing a decathlon. The finish line was visible, but the unsympathetic terrain just would not let us get there. We must have stopped the car two dozen times in this last stretch. It was literal torture, for both Landon and us. However, we made it and we swore we would never make a trip like that again in this lifetime.

After a few months of settling in, I finally got tired of running in place. I got on the computer and looked up biomedical doctors in the state of Florida. If I never believed in fate before this moment, I did now. Dr. Jerry Kartzinel MD, a doctor I remember reading about in Jenny McCarthy's book "Louder than Words" was practicing in the state of Florida. Coincidentally, he was next on my list of biomedical doctors to try. Further down the road, I discovered Dr. Kartzinel co-authored a book with Jenny McCarthy called "Healing and Preventing Autism", a New York Times Bestseller. I found this book to be a much easier read and less technical than Dr. Bock's, but thoroughly enjoyed reading both. Not only was Dr. Kartzinel in Florida, he was in Orlando; a hop, skip, and jump away. Interesting, because I thought for sure he practiced in California. As it turned out, he practiced in both states. I'm not a big believer in accidents; I considered this a well-deserved twist of fate. My life has always proven to turn strange paranormal corners like this. I am being completely sincere when I tell you we literally picked a place on the map and ended up in the same vicinity as the next doctor we were going to call. He was meant to be our doctor and I could barely wait to pick up the phone. Dr. Kartzinel's receptionist and staff were super friendly. The wait time to get an appointment was not bad at all, and we did not feel treated as just a number. The office instructed us to bring all past lab work/paperwork from previous doctors with us to the appointment, and to make sure we were on time.

11

SUPERHERO

As our race against time was closing in, the window to save Landon grew smaller inside my head. The element of time was crucial, and the longer we waited, the worse off it would be for him. As luck would have it, we knew we had found the right doctor for Landon, as our journey would end with him.

I do not often compliment others, even when they deserve it. I reserve special judgment for people I have no words for. I believe Dr. Kartzinel is a superhero. He knows he has a big responsibility in life, and like the superhero Spiderman, "with great powers comes great responsibility". They are rarely shown gratitude, and never arrogant. Here he was, arriving at the scene of a very horrible accident to save a life. I'm sure it's difficult emotionally for him to see injured children come through his door day after day.

He was a man devoted to his work and altogether displayed competence, confidence, leadership, and he incorporated something no other doctor I have seen has had...humor. It is an astounding and integral characteristic, and believe me; it can go a long way. It's very important to feel and look at someone this way when they hold your child's life in their hands. It allows you to trust them. Had he not owned these qualities, it would have been just another dead end for us. His quality attributes bled into his staff as well, always encouraging questions and phone calls. What I liked most about this office was the individualized attention and how they made us feel right at home. We were never surrounded by the chaos of other patients, always making sure you are the only ones coming in before the visit, and the only ones leaving when the appointment is over. It is completely stress free for everyone involved. I'm not sure if this process is done to make it easier on the child or the parents! His son David, who works as the office manager, assured us we could call them 60 times a day if we had to. This is no exaggeration, I promise you. I am willing to bet a lot of uneasy, overwhelmed parents of autistic children probably do call 60 times a day, especially when new treatment plans are thrown at them. With Dr. C and Bock, I wanted to call every five minutes. The accessible lines of communication and open arms were just a few of many things that really set Dr. Kartzinel and his staff apart from the rest. We liked them from day one.

Like Groundhog Day, we told our story once more from beginning to the end, and yes, we would have to get another blood draw. These blood draws by themselves were going to send me over the edge. He put us at ease and explained there are mobile phlebotomists we could call who come to your home and draw the blood there. That way Landon would be comfortable and not stressed out. This may work! As far as the cost of the blood work goes, it turned out to be only a fraction of what Bock's blood draw would have cost us. After getting this out of the way, he reprimanded me about making assumptions. I assumed it was my fault Landon was in the condition he was in and told him why. He quickly shot down my theory about the yeast infection causing all the problems and suggested maybe I should stay off the internet. (I never did comply...I continue to look everything up). I was so sure this was my doing, but he was quick to explain there was more science and factors behind it than this, and although maybe yeast could have been a contributing factor, I should not jump to any conclusions.

The appointment was drawing to a close, but I was not done by a long shot. As usual, I needed to know the answers to everything about Landon right then and there. I peppered Dr. Kartzinel with my routine doctor interrogation drill, consisting of questions he needed to answer that ranged from the present moment to Landon's teenage years. In the midst of this, Dr. Kartzinel calmly responded with a rather astute answer I never could erase from my mind. "I am just trying to get him to kindergarten, woman!" And this is what would become our primary goal, an extremely time sensitive one. Knowing the early years were the most important when it came to reversing autism, we ended the excuses that day. He was so right, we needed to focus on taking one step at a time. First and foremost, that first step would be the lab work right in front of us.

Part of the blood draw would be testing for that MTHFR gene mutation, which he said comes from Ed's side of the family. I remember him asking about our ethnic backgrounds and mentioning how Italians are poor methylators. As it turns out, Ed is mostly Italian. That is quite interesting because now that I think about it, a lot of people I know who have autistic children are of Italian descent. Out of curiosity, in the future I always

made it a point to ask parents whose children have spectrum issues if they have Italian ancestry in their blood. To rehash what I
said earlier, if a large majority of autistic kids do have the
MTHFR mutation, it makes me wonder just how many of these
kids can be helped by B12 alone? It saddens me to think about all
the parents who are never alerted to something that can make
such a big difference.

Landon would get tested for allergies (IGG and IGE), lipid
panel, along with a complete metabolic panel test. At this time,
the only supplements we were giving him were B12 shots, cod
liver oil, pro EFA, coconut kefir, and oxy powder to cleanse the
bowels and intestines. We described our situation to the doctor
the best we could. Recounting the pileup of additional symptoms
was difficult because with each new doctor, we had to start from
the beginning. That meant recalling each new symptom four
times from beginning to end, and trying to get him to incorporate the significance of the positive milestones as well. Here was
our summary up to this point.

Here was our summary up to this point: Landon's language
skills were made up of mostly two word sentences which were
very hard to understand. Sometimes he just made sounds, incomprehensible to everyone. Behavior wise, he would play on the
iPad all day and was rigidly stuck on routines. Earlier, I mentioned OCD behaviors he exhibited during regression, and more
he had accumulated since then. He would not let me drive the
car, only Ed. He had to have his toys in a certain way or he would
have a meltdown that would last anywhere from 15 minutes to
hours. He awoke several times a night soaking two to three diapers. His diet consisted of pureed turnips, rutabaga, beets,
broccoli, cauliflower, and fermented sauerkraut. His diapers
smelled like a decomposed rodent, his pores emitted a putrid
odor, and his belly was distended. Landon would occasionally

bang his head during those man-on-fire episodes and sometimes push his brother down. Also very disturbing was that he was unable to climb the stairs. I thought maybe he was just being difficult and wanted to be carried everywhere but as Dr. Kartzinel later explained from the blood work, he had no energy. I attributed this to his extremely low blood sugar/broken triangle (unable to gather and release energy), and thought it was likely the cause of Landon almost fainting many times at the playground or even in his chair at mealtimes.

Prior to going to this appointment with Dr. Kartzinel, both Ed and I still held out hope Landon was not autistic, mostly due to two reasons. Not only was autism something we had pictured entirely different in our minds, but secondly, we were never told straight out he was autistic. That is until we saw the diagnosis sheet with autism typed at the very top of Dr. Kartzinel's report. Every behavior up to this point had a justification behind it or we excused it as something he would eventually outgrow after treating the yeast. Even though we knew biomedical doctors treated autism, we really sought help here because we knew he could treat Landon's issues characteristic to that of autistic children (leaky gut/candida). We knew in the back of our minds there was a large possibility he was autistic, but outwardly denied it until the day we landed in Dr. Kartzinel's office. Landon never had the thousand-yard stare I ignorantly attributed to autism. I did picture this level of autism as a place Landon would have ended up a year down the road, had we not gotten him biomedical help. Ed and I never spoke about the diagnosis; we always dealt with it silently and kept to ourselves. We never told anyone in our family circle Landon was autistic either, not because we were ashamed of it, rather, we did not want to feel sorry for ourselves. I never felt it was relevant, especially considering we were intent on turning it around. Besides, with all the grief forced upon us, nobody earned the right to know. Who would understand anyway? Wasn't this just another label assignment? Again, all just wasted breath. They had not walked in our shoes so how would they ever truly understand? They will just have to wait until they read the book.

Based on our input and his analysis, Dr. Kartzinel's assessment, tests, and blood labs of Landon (age 3-4) looked something like this. (Some of the supplements you see in the next chapter were already part of our treatment plan but the new ones we were excited to try. Also, many of them were retracted during treatment.)

Assessment

Autism, Repetitive behaviors, Routine oriented,
Fixations, Communication delay, Social delay,
Sleep: dysfunctional, multiple night awakenings,
Distended abdomen, Language delay,
Toileting: won't initiate, but will go,
Anxiety over not getting something he wants

Diagnostic Tests

Comp Metabolic Panel, CBC, Lipid, Vitamin D,
25 Hydroxy, FERRITIN, MTHFR DNA,
C-Reactive Protein, IGE,
SED Rate ELISA 96 IGG Food Panel w/o wellness

Before seeing Dr. Kartzinel, we were already using cod liver oil, kefir, and B12 injections off and on. Other supplements he started Landon on were:

Vitamin A – 1 drop per day, Cod Liver Oil – 1 tsp,
Liquid Iron – 1 tsp 2x per day,
Prescription Leucovorin (folic acid) – ½ pill 2x per day,
PS Caps (for adrenals) – ½ capsule 2x per day,

Liquid calcium/magnesium – 1 tsp 2x per day,
Vitamin E – 1 capsule 2x per day,
Vitamin D3 – 2 drops per day,
Ester Vitamin C – ½ capsule 2x per day,
DMG – 1 ml 2x per day – helps metabolism process,
B12 injections – .05 ml = 1250 mcg every other day,
Continue with coconut kefir, probiotics, and keep
going with the diet.
Other possible yeast killers: Grapefruit seed extract,
pau d'arco

Landon was deficient in a lot of these supplements while others boosted his immune system.

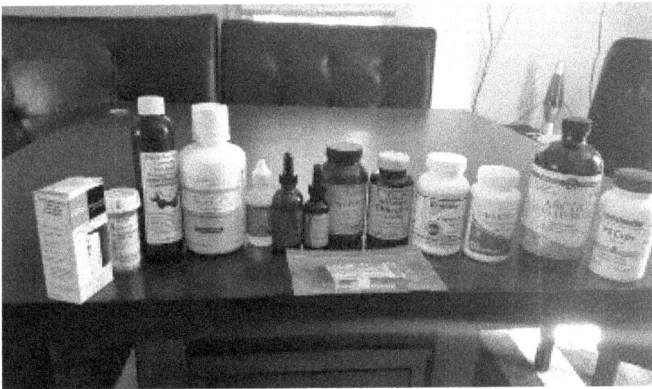

Supplements we use now

12

BLOOD DRAW

Finding a mobile phlebotomist was much easier than we had thought. A lab down the road from us had one that mostly went to senior citizens' residences, but were happy to come to ours. We braced ourselves for the worst that day, and even prepared a beach blanket to wrap him up in if we needed stabilization. Ed was confident we could pull this off without traumatizing Landon. We decided the draw would be in the living room, in front of the TV where Landon felt comfortable. I held Cole in my room while the phlebotomist stayed in the living room battle zone. He was absolutely amazing. This man was somehow able to keep Landon calm the entire time, with not even a peep of protest arising from that room. He could not find a vein in his arm that could support the needle so he eventually drew all the blood from the top of Landon's hand. The whole ordeal went off without a hitch in about 30 minutes time. It was the work of a divine being. Saying very little, he arrived and left quickly, disappearing like an angel into the night. Only an angel could have pulled off a phenomenon such as this. All the blood was successfully drawn; totaling about seven to eight tubes. It felt like the weight of the world was lifted from our shoulders. This had caused a lot of stress for us in the past because treatment really cannot begin without the diagnostics tests. We were never able to get it all done until now. In the past, so much of our anxiety and despair had to do with not knowing what was wrong or what was crucially needed to make him better. Now we would know, and had an excellent doctor that could explain it to us in detail. With that out of the way, we stuck to the kefir and waited for the results to come back. This is what followed:

Plan (all added after blood analysis)
Cholesterol is low – concern about cholesterol
Creon 3000 one with each meal

Thyroid
TSH (indicator of thyroid function) is 4.8 and should be under 2
Max Thyroid ½ capsule daily

Iron
OTC "FERRITIN" or fer-in-sol 1 ml twice daily

Elevated HISTADINE
5HTP 100 mg twice daily
Vitamin C raise to 500mg twice daily
B6 50 mg one daily

Language
  Vayarin 2 caps daily
  PHOSPHALINE ½ tsp twice daily

Allergies
  Zyrtec (replaced with Quercitin supplement)
  Singulair

For excessive sweating consider MSM (sulpher)
Antibiotic to treat a bacteria found in his stool

To our surprise, we noticed not all were supplements. Dr. Kartzinel included medications such as Zyrtec and Singulair (allergies), Max Thyroid (thyroid), Creon (cholesterol) and Vayerin (language) to which Ed and I were both opposed. Based on past experiences I have had with allergy medications for my asthma, I will tell anyone it only caused my asthma to become worse when I used it. We did not tell Dr. Kartzinel right away that we planned on opting out of the allergy medications (he replaced with natural Quercitin anyway), but later decided to express our concerns to him. Also, to be fair to him we did decide to give them a try. He explained the medications only served a short-term purpose, as he wanted little to no side effects. His motto was "minimal intervention for the maximum result". This "integrative" part of the treatment is where the lines became a bit blurred for us. Like the allergy medications, we tried most of these medications but ultimately stopped due to reactions Landon had with some, and also because of fear on our part. We had to be hyper-alert about what he ingested because of his leaky gut, therefore some prescriptions were scary for us. It was no surprise when we were told a certain antibiotic could trigger a two year regression for some kids. On the other side of the coin, the prescriptions for the subcutaneous B12 and Leucovorin were life saving, so I cannot say all prescription medications were negative.

Ed and I were birds of a feather, instinctually repelled by prescription medications. In this case, just as with life in general, we always follow our instincts. Who knows, maybe these medications could have saved us months of healing time and brought us to the finish line sooner rather than later, with little to no side effects. I believe that was Dr. Kartzinel's ultimate reasoning. We finally came clean with him one day regarding our fears. He understood and gave me a good example regarding this issue. His position was, as long as there are no major side effects, sometimes taking the pharmaceutical route is more beneficial. "If you had a yeast infection, would you rather have it over with in one shot with a prescription or would you rather cure it naturally and have it take weeks or months?" He made a very valid point! Having a yeast infection is not a pleasant experience, so my bet is most women would opt for the prescription and be rid of it. (Dr. Kartzinel also happened to use as an example one of the only conditions I would choose prescription medication over a natural one!) Had the doctors given us the antifungals to begin with, maybe the man-on-fire episodes would have only lasted a few weeks and not a year and a half. Stubborn as we were, we still opted to take the long route. As Ed and I recall from "The Tortoise and the Hare", slow and steady won the race. We knew we would still get to the finish line first. For every prescription medication, there had to be an alternative. We decided to nix some of the pharmaceuticals and see if we could improve things naturally, which we would find out when it came time for the next round of blood work.

I was surprised, but happy to hear Landon had no chronic inflammation going on. Landon's metabolic profile of his liver, kidney, and salts from this blood work were normal. His lipid profile (cholesterol level) was terrifyingly low. Dr. K explained cholesterol is important for hormone production. Since Landon was not producing hormones, we had to give him cholesterol. Our first order of business was trying something called Sonic Cholesterol, two capsules twice daily. This turned out to be short-lived. Initially, we had tried this supplement with Dr. Bock, but it did not go over well. Again, we saw a high level of irritability after trying this multiple times, possibly due to a preservative. Our only option now would be loads of natural fats like coconut and avocado oils.

HYPOTHYROIDISM

Landon's adrenal readings told us he was in adrenal distress and at an abnormal level. I recall an entire week of Ben's show dedicated to adrenals and cortisol. The distress Landon had was causing signals to be sent from his brain to his adrenal glands, resulting in cortisol being released into the blood. Ben describes cortisol as a stress management hormone which meant Landon's body was under an exorbitant amount of chronic stress. The doctor mentioned Landon had hypothyroidism, which meant Landon's thyroid was not functioning well, and not producing enough hormones. Remember the triangle Ben talks about? This is the adrenal thyroid area, the third and final point of the triangle to malfunction...the crux of what I believed to be Landon's impending immune system breakdown. We were at the point of the triangle Ben calls the jumping off point, where chronic degenerative disease sets in, whatever it may be. Verbatim, Ben explains hypothyroidism as either "primary (immune system attack on the thyroid following leaky gut syndrome), or secondary to adrenal gland dysfunction." Ben states that in both cases of primary and secondary hypothyroidism, adrenal weakness needs to be undertaken. No question in my mind this was primary and would not have surfaced as a health issue if Landon had a properly functioning digestive system. Hypothyroidism, he says, is the point where all major disease sets in. This is not about mind over matter...you cannot fight any disease without a healthy functioning thyroid. At this juncture it was critical for us to turn things around. Being that Landon's hypothyroidism was primary following leaky gut syndrome, supplementing his thyroid was not going to be good enough. We had to fix his gut! Thinking about this in terms of a military threat, his body was now at Defcon 1 where the threat (disease) was imminent and could strike at anytime. I confirmed with Ben on his show that you cannot get a chronic degenerative disease before arriving at the "jumping off" point of the triangle. (The Bright Side March 7, 2018, I am the first caller of the day. If you would like more information about the Triangle of Disease, please listen regularly to his show as it's often a topic of discussion.) This really worried me, because if all chronic degenerative diseases set in at the hypothyroidism stage, he must be in the worst trouble imaginable. I try not to think about what was around the corner for Landon had we not intervened when we did. It also made complete sense now about his lack of energy and why he was always on the verge of passing out. If I am interpreting Ben correctly, Landon's malfunctioning thyroid that followed his blood sugar breakdown made it impossible to allocate energy, which is what the process of the third point of the triangle is responsible for. Decrypting Landon's health in relation to Ben's triangle of disease outline is what would be my wake up call. Now was no time for worry, it was time for action.

REPAIRING THE TRIANGLE AND TELEGRAPH LINE
PS CAPS, IODINE, ZINC, VITAMINS B AND D

Now is a good time to introduce Ben and Dr. Kartzinel, our "telegraph line repairman". On top of the physical challenges, we needed to change how the messages coming in were being processed going out. Notice how all points on Ben's Triangle of Disease were affected with Landon, and how Dr. Kartzinel was addressing all areas of the triangle: the gut, the adrenal thyroid, and blood sugar. Believe it or not, it all tied together. Taking a step back, I noticed everything fell into place. I saw the break-down of all three infrastructure points of this triangle with Landon, in exactly the order Ben described. I am willing to bet autistic children need to be repaired at every point of this Triangle of Disease. At the very least I am sure it would improve their overall condition. I need to point out that for most people the triangle breakdown occurs over the course of their lifetime, whereas for Landon the three point breakdown all occurred by age three. For us we had one focus: to supplement and repair. If we could fix Landon up in all those sectors, his neurological and physical health will be back on track. Bringing Ben and Dr. Kartzinel together like this to illustrate these points makes it so worth it! (They are whom I consider to be the more health conscious Ben & Jerry!)

Supplements on Landon's menu included PS capsules, which stands for phosphatidylserine. According to Dr. Kartzinel, these capsules would help stabilize him in the cortisol area (high anxiety), reducing stress, and improving brain function. Along with PS capsules for adrenals, we planned on supplementing him naturally with B, D, and C vitamins, zinc, and large quantities of dried seaweed and himalayan/celtic sea salts to support his thyroid. Initially, Landon's first blood panel with Dr. C suggested he needed iodine. We did try nascent iodine which travels directly to the thyroid. His reaction was characteristic of the distinguishable die-off, most likely due to a dozen things happening to him at once, so we backed off. Knowing Landon was deficient in iodine and aware essential vitamins and minerals are not associated with allergic reactions, I look back now with regret. I take this supplement now and have felt the effects. I will be supplementing Landon with iodine in the nascent form again, as opposed to potassium iodide. Hopefully this is something I will be able to get everyone in my family on board with.

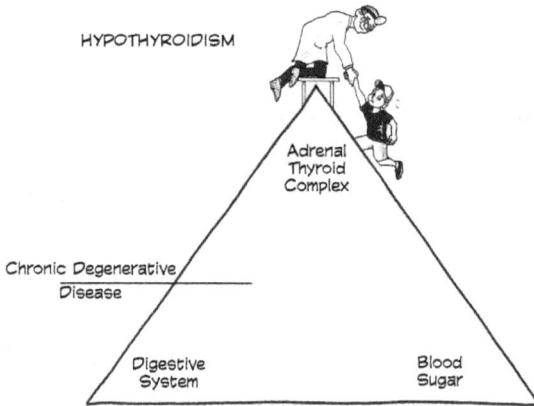

IRON

Next up on the lab report was Landon's iron level. His level measured a 23, whereas normally it should be a 63. Dr. K went on to say iron is responsible for red blood cell function as well as cognitive function. We were to administer Ferritin liquid iron three teaspoons a day.

VITAMIN D

Next we moved on to Vitamin D. Vitamin D levels of a normal person should be 80-100, but Landon's measured only 17. We were to administer two drops a day on food ASAP.

DMG

Dimethylglycine (DMG) assists metabolism, immune system and brain health. We would give Landon 1 ml 2x/day. (If our heads were not spinning at this point from all the supplements, it would soon start.)

IGG/IGE

Next on the list was IGG and IGE – a measure of how allergic he was to the world. We already knew Landon had one major anaphylactic IGE allergy to peanuts. The rest of his allergies were really intolerances which we intended on reversing. Below 60 is normal and Landon's read at 1323. We were not surprised to hear this, we already knew he was allergic to the world based on how messed up his digestive system was and how far advanced his leaky gut had become. I believe Dr. Kartzinel had maybe seen levels this high only a few times, his clinic high being just over 7,000. Incredibly, he was able to correct that patient's level back down to normal numbers. As far as food allergy tests were concerned, I was unimpressed. Divided up into allergy, stool and urine, and blood, each were sent to different labs for analysis. The allergy reports that came back were completely off. For example, the test said that among other things, Landon was allergic to red apples, red grapes, blueberries, and blackberries. These were all fruits we had been giving him for quite some time based on trial and error. It said all green fruits like green apples, green grapes, and kiwi he was not allergic to. So we decided to swap the fruits for a week and see what happened. We fed him the green fruits and laid off the ones we normally gave him. Little sensitivity rashes appeared on his backside immediately afterwards. Besides the green apples (we always gave him those), everything else we switched to caused a skin reaction. Did they go down a list and choose food allergies randomly? I never gave much credibility to allergy tests based on my experience and this just confirmed what I already believed. This was not a reflection on Dr. Kartzinel, he had no involvement with what the lab concluded. I just believe food allergy testing in general is inconclusive.

B12 (Methylcobalamin/Leucovorin)

As suspected, Landon did have the faulty gene, MTHFR (methylenetetrahydrofolate), passed on from Ed. Dr. Kartzinel explained in detail that it is responsible for methylation of every cell. I know I wrote about this earlier but Dr. Kartzinel's explanation is the easiest to understand. He broke his explanation down and I noted it as simply as I could. MTHFR is designed to make glutathione, a natural antioxidant and chelator. Since Landon's methylation is dysfunctional, he cannot secrete or methylate toxins as efficiently as most of us can every day of our lives. In this area, Landon was given one good gene (me) and one bad (Ed). I liked this metaphor he used to explain it rather rudimentary. Imagine Landon as a car factory that cranks out 100 cars per day. But instead of cranking out 100 cars a day, Landon cranks out 63. He is not as efficient compared to those with normal gene expression. The B12 paired with leucovorin (folinic acid) would be essential for helping this process along. I remember Dr. Kartzinel later referring to the B12 as "happy juice". This analogy was 100% accurate and fitting. He could not have come up with a better description if he tried. (I will explain in further detail how this change came about later on.)

When pregnant with Landon, I recall being told I had a one in three chance of giving birth to a child with Down Syndrome. They based this on blood work and specific tests. I cannot help but wonder, since Landon does not have Down Syndrome, if the MTHFR somehow threw the test off and they read that mutation instead? It's a silly notion I know, but the doctors seemed quite surprised Landon did not have Down Syndrome when he was born. Another reason I say this is because my neighbor Karen has a nine year old son with Down Syndrome, according to her doctor's diagnosis. She told me she never believed it was Down Syndrome, she always believed it was autism. I had to agree with her after seeing him. He did not have the features of a Down Syndrome child at all, and those features are usually very distinguishable. Again, maybe the test was thrown off by the MTHFR defect that her child might have instead, and he was really just misdiagnosed. If that's the case, she can very possibly turn things around. I told her everything I knew, including our doctor information, hoping she would get on top of this pronto.

CALCIUM/MAGNESIUM

Liquid calcium magnesium was the next supplement Landon needed. He was not getting any calcium because he could not drink dairy. I was afraid of this supplement because I thought it had caused problems in the past with Dr. Bock's program. Landon's reaction was once again off the wall, but instead of stopping this time we would re-introduce calcium at a lower level and build up.

ANTIBIOTIC

Concerning the antibiotic, I can see how someone reading this could make an argument that using one was contradictory, seeing that this is what contributed to the whole debacle to begin with. But to Dr. Kartzinel's defense, sometimes they are necessary. As long as we continued to feed Landon's gut with probiotics, killing bacteria that were found in his stool with antibiotics could make way for huge progressions.

Meanwhile, our routine still consisted of daily trips to Whole Foods Market for his dietary needs. We made sure everything was organic and nothing processed. Cutting up the rutabaga, boiling, then pureeing it several times a week was breaking Ed's back. It was laborious but necessary. Eventually we rotated this out with other vegetables as Landon's digestion grew stronger. We eventually progressed to 8 tablespoons a day of coconut kefir, four in the morning and four in the afternoon. Taking Landon anywhere in public during this time was not even contemplated. Although the healing reactions were less frequent, they were just too unpredictable.

I decided to be brave one day, and took both of my little ones to the library. I'm not sure what I was thinking, maybe because Landon's reactions were becoming less severe and I wanted to feel like a normal mother taking her children places. Landon seemed to play calmly for the first hour, but when it came time to leave, forget it. I remember having to put one child under each arm, while running out to the car before we became a spectacle. Only a few stopped to watch the show, more in amusement rather than empathy. That's the difference with me. Anytime I witness a mother in this type of similar situation, I immediately recognize she needs help. I'm not talking about "let me help you with the door", I'm talking more about "let me help you gather your wits and guide you through this long battle ahead of you".

Most of my life I had a "not my problem" attitude, but now life had turned the tables and decided to throw me a curve ball. I learned real fast that not only is this my problem now, it is my full-time job. Something inside me definitely changed, as I now consider it my goal and my obligation to help any parent going through what we did, overcome the obstacles. Along with my newly acquired sense of empathy, intervening was something I felt had now been assigned to me. Sometimes in passing, I watch and wonder just how close these parents are to the edge. Would they step back from the edge if they knew help existed? Sometimes it's more than saving autistic children, it's also about saving their parents. The problem with this is approaching an unapproachable parent. I don't think initializing the conversation with, "Hi, it appears your child is autistic. I would like to help you." will go very far. Different kinds of people require different approaches. Once you accomplish the initial nosy introduction, whether it be at the mall or grocery store, you have to find a way to capture their attention and get them to absorb the information in five minutes or less. I will drop everything and approach a parent in need of help if I think they will listen. However, in this endeavor I have discovered a lot of parents do not want help and have learned to accept their child's condition as permanent and unfixable, which may be true in a lot of cases.

GOLD COINS TO A CAT

Take my friends Preston, Sam, and John my roofer (I am changing names to protect identities). Preston and Sam both have two autistic children and John has an autistic granddaughter (two of them full Italian heritage). They have been my most frustrating obstacles I have encountered yet. On multiple occasions I have tried convincing them not to accept their children's autism as hopeless, even offering to accompany them to a biomedical doctor's office of their choice. I gave them the name of Landon's doctor, told them about diet, supplements, the gut connection, and how far we had come. I told John I would pay for his granddaughter's initial treatment visit. She was older now and maybe too far gone, (20's or 30's) but his stories about the medications she was doped up on made me want to take action. He told me he believed all the medications on top of one another caused her to develop lupus. I cannot say I agree with that but I'm sure the medications were not helping to heal her condition. Ultimately, he blamed his daughter for backing out, so they never went for an office visit. I finally became tired of making this my problem. I was swimming upstream with him and finally realized I was fighting a losing battle trying to help.

In Preston's case, no sooner do I finish telling him about changing his kids' diet, he is changing the subject (as if the television show "The Good Doctor" was a better topic of interest). Unbelievably, I'm suggesting to him a way out of this, a possible key to unlock his children's universe, and he shuts down as soon as he hears about eliminating sugar and carbohydrates. He wants no part in it. Something Preston did not get is the irony that healing his children could potentially be more miraculous than the Hollywood television series he references regarding a young autistic surgeon.

Then there's Sam, who thinks it's too late for his children. His kids are now teenagers, and just trying to get this past his ex-wife would be impossible to begin with. As he tells it, she has given up holding out for hope and would never go for this. He mentioned how they tried every treatment known in the past, but to no avail. I'm really wondering if they went the biomedical route, or was it through a mainstream "autism specialist"? Regardless, I know they all heard me, but not one listened. It's incomprehensible why they wouldn't be jumping all over this information I gave them. Maybe they thought the path was too burdensome and accepting the condition is easier than doing the work. Or they believe I am full of it. As sacred as this information was to me, it was as useless to them as gold coins to a cat. I know I, as a parent, would never stop looking for answers.

13

I KNOW

"Those of you who know will always know, and those of you who don't, will never. There is no changing the mind of those who would dance before the golden idol. There is no way to ever change them. They will not change." - Michael Savage

I have come to learn that some people just have the ability to see. Ed and I always agreed that some people get it and some do not. "It" could mean anything, but my definition of "it" pertains to whatever the truth happens to be. "It" was our constant theme while hurdling through this trek. When you go through tumultuous times, sometimes you may feel alone. You may feel this way because mainstream society does not always accept your beliefs. Just as the saying goes, "the nail that sticks out gets hammered down." If you choose to seek biomedical treatment for your child, you may not get reinforcements from anyone but yourselves, and success may only be accomplished through your own dedication and will. Family or friends may turn on you and make you feel as if you are doing the wrong thing for your child. You may get bullied along the way, whether it is by pediatricians, schools, friends, or family. In the end, if you heal your child, none of it will matter. The important thing for Ed and I was to be a strong team. We persisted through the nonsense and the garbage dished at us from every direction whether it was a pediatrician hell-bent on using intimidation tactics for not vaccinating our child, our own parents insisting we were crazy or just comments from the ignorant general public. Your greatest ally is your spouse/partner. It is my belief that support you draw from each other is where you will find the greatest strength. Trying to explain this or any biomedical dialogue to the average Joe is futile and I recommend not wasting a minute of your breath unless it is for assistance purposes.

During this difficult time both my parents made independent visits. Not to pick on them, but I mention them throughout this book for a reason. I believe they represent a large majority of the preconditioned population, especially regarding those who are uninformed and quick to judge. Neither was sympathetic to what was happening around us and neither offered any emotional support. The doctors we had seen up to this point were referred to as "quacks", (in my opinion, a pre-conditioned term often used to refer to doctors who use alternative treatment methods and used to sway the public in another direction), and Landon was nothing more than a discipline problem. We were catering to his every whim and demand he had, and we were thus creating a monster. At other times they insinuated we were subjecting Landon to intolerable conditions with this treatment plan we had him on. Whatever the criticism was, it fell directly upon us. We were told straight out we were failures as parents. Landon had been at the pinnacle of his distress and had meltdowns the entire visit from my dad, who insisted on instilling his own strict verbal punishments on Landon. Not heeding our warning to stop yelling at Landon for his behavior, my dad was finally kicked out of the house one day by Ed. I walked into the kitchen as the commotion topped out, and noticed Ed pointing to the door. In the years I have known him, I had never heard Ed raise his voice, until that day.

Not one person from the outside, especially my parents, was able to understand Landon could not help or control what was happening to him. He could not process food in his gut or messages to and from his brain; his telegraph line was broken. The last thing we needed from people who are supposed to lend a hand in times like this is to be called idiots or failures. We had a code red medical crisis going on, and drowning with no life raft, right in front of their eyes. When we tried to come up for air, instead of extending a hand, they pushed our heads under water. Throughout our ordeal, their primary focus was the condition of the house and the messy bathrooms. Lost in the calamity of Landon's nosedive, we let the condition of the house deteriorate and they were sure to let us know. The disapproval extended to Landon's diet which was criticized from day one. "Oh he'll be fine, give him the pizza, eggs, the bowl of sukiyaki…he wants to eat it. You are starving your child." Yeah, we tried that once or twice, and he projectile vomited for three hours. During our treatment, my parents would give him forbidden foods at family gatherings and we were left to clean up the vomit as well as help his gut recover from the setback this had most likely created. At night Landon would wake up hallucinating most likely due to the toxins from these foods circulating through his system. Nobody except Ed and I dealt with these downsides, it always fell on us. Nothing in my life was more infuriating than people who do not get it, and insisted on asserting their own opinions upon our lives.

Fortunately for us, Dr. Kartzinel was our biggest ally. He had our backs and we had his. He carried a firm "stand your ground" position and encouraged us to do exactly that. In fact, he solemnly told us to have anyone call him at anytime and he will explain biologically what is going on. He could communicate better than anyone why Landon could not function like the rest of us. It was such a relief to have him at ringside. I cannot emphasize enough the respect, the admiration, and the love I have for this man. I don't say this just because he was saving our son, but because of his commitment to the cause, and the understanding of the annoyances that went along with it. Our problems were his problems too. As the only one who stood in our corner, it was a blessing he was intelligent, fluent, and had the certitude to stand firm in his work. Maybe what we were doing was against our parents' beliefs, but we knew we were saving our son's life. Dr. Kartzinel was firmly a hero to us. He proved time and again he would step in as our voice and defend us at anytime if needed. He was our only advocate in this race.

Landon needed our attention, we were not spoiling him. If he screamed to be held 24/7, then that is what we had to do to get through this. He was healing, and he needed us more than ever. I must admit in the beginning even I questioned this babying treatment he had us accustomed to. Ed held strong to his beliefs and was the one who really enforced this, designating himself to hold Landon all night when he screamed bloody murder.

At times I found Ed asleep on the floor next to Landon's bed holding his hand, doing this when Landon was a baby too. A lot of pediatricians in the past recommended we put him to bed and shut the door, let him cry. Ed believed from day one and convinced me as well, that Landon was a different situation and required different measures. We must be there round-the-clock for this child. If he cries to be held you hold him, no if's, and's, or but's. He is sick and a sick child needs you. A lot of the catering had to do with avoiding a meltdown; because once it started there was no going back. But mostly we accommodated him because he was ill. We held him when he wanted (when he let me), carried him, lie next to him, and let him have his routine for as long as it took. When Landon was about a year old, I remember he and Ed were in a car accident. Ed's airbag went off and Landon went bananas (they were both uninjured). When I got to the scene, Landon would not even let me hold him, only Ed. As a mother, this really hits you hard. It was then I realized I had lost him in some way. Now almost three, Landon was getting older and growing more demanding. Ed's hair was falling out and his weight had drastically dropped either due to stress or because Landon would not allow him to eat or do anything not involving complete attention to him. It was not what I would call a healthy weight loss. When I mentioned earlier about Ed relinquishing his rights as a free man, this is what I was talking about. Although we had our roles taking care of the kids, the burden fell more heavily on Ed and this was something that had to change.

14

LIGHT AT THE END OF THE TUNNEL

In the beginning stages of this new treatment plan (Landon was three), we decided to enroll Landon in a PPK. (pre-preschool) Since we had somehow miraculously potty trained him, what better time than the present? We thought it would also be a good idea to get him acclimated to other kids and learn to socialize, not just with his brother. We made this decision because of a few positive changes, even though his tantrums were still off the wall.

One of the changes I am referring to took place just outside our pool area. It was by far my favorite memorable moment, and it absolutely blew me away. This was the day I knew that if we held out hope, everything was going to turn out alright. As Ed and I stood talking with our friend Daniel in the lanai, I looked up to see our youngest one, Cole, start walking towards the pool.

Before I could react, I see Landon rush over and place himself between his little brother and the pool, as if to block him from going any further. When Cole tried to go around him, Landon would move accordingly to stay between his brother and the pool. I could not believe my eyes; I was witnessing some sort of breakthrough! He was being protective. He recognized the potential danger of his brother falling into the pool. Does an autistic kid do this, or was it a sign of recovery? I was so proud of him at that moment! I began going over in my head what new supplement could possibly be responsible for this behavior. Truthfully, I believe it was the beginning of the end for the toxins leaving his body.

After this incident, I was left with a very odd yet comforting feeling I would never have to worry about Cole falling into the pool with Landon around. Who would believe the day would come where Landon was the one watching out for others? Well, it was definitely a sign for better things to come. He made other leaps in progress, such as talking more, and answering questions with "yeah" or "uh-huh" instead of repeating the last words of the question. He also asked "what's that noise" and "too loud" when the workmen were hammering down the carpet. One day his little brother was crying. Landon walked upstairs and knelt down next to him. I almost fell over in my chair as he softly said "Ohhh Cole, why you cry?" If we had never witnessed some of what we called "miraculous breakthroughs" of the kefir, or the aloe, or any of the supplements, we would have stayed far away from them. These were signs of recovery, and we were sticking with what was working.

High points and funny moments always kept us hopeful. For several weeks, we were unaware Landon had been helping his little brother escape out of his crib. We had followed him one day after hearing pleas for help from his brother after putting him down for a nap. We watched as Landon pushed the desk chair over to the crib so Cole could climb out. Again, not the typical thought process of an autistic child. One more instance similar to this, was one day he needed to reach something that was sitting high on top of the refrigerator. He put four different objects next to each other, each one a little bit taller than the other allowing him to ultimately climb onto the highest level to reach his target. Another sign materialized one day after a tirade from losing a toy car. Landon turned to Ed and said "Dad, green truck mom's van." He wanted his favorite green Hulk truck! On a separate occasion he asked, "What number is this?" He used the word "what"...his communication skills were flourishing! While making his lunch the following week, Landon spilled his licorice tea all over the floor and pouted. A thought occurred to me at this moment. Do autistic kids pout? I'm really not sure. I asked him for a hug, and he ran over and gave me a huge hug. This was the beginning of showing affection, just more confirmation to help me see that he was improving. His brain was functioning, and the lights were on inside. We had to keep doing what we were doing.

I'm sure parents with kids who develop at a normal level, never catch themselves jumping on each and every word their child says, but this was a miracle to us. Funny when events like this happen, it takes us by surprise. We wait all day for him to do it again, but he never does. By the end of the day we have ourselves convinced it was a fluke and maybe he never said anything at all, and it was just our imagination. Elation, then reality, exhilarating highs, and dreadful lows. The next minute turns on a dime.

Enduring the volume of Landon's screams sometimes required special measures. One time, Ed grabbed my big headphones to drown out the screaming. Landon would not let him elude his hollering as he shouted, "No bubblehead! No bubblehead!". The headphones must have looked like big bubbles on Ed's ears for which he showed displeasure. Although it was not funny at the time, we can now look back and chuckle. Sometimes you just have to laugh to keep yourself sane, and this was one of those moments.

Before PPK, I had to fill out a Diagnostic Learning Resources system form. They would contact us for an appointment, and they would also test Landon and see if he needed IEP (Individual Education Program). On the day of Landon's pre-K assessment, we abstained from giving him any supplements. We wanted him on his best behavior for this assessment, although looking back I'm not sure this was the best idea considering his good behavior was not typical for him, and this evaluation was to place him in a preschool setting best suited for his capacity. I know giving him supplements at all sounds illogical at this point, because it leads one to think; if it's causing all this bad behavior, why do it? This is where I like to use the pendulum analogy. It swings a little forward then backward, then forward more, and then backward even more, etc. It sure did seem like it was weighed more heavily towards backwards most of the time. The point is, I would much rather experience the bad behavior and see him improve, than have him act tranquil and plateau. However, there was no denying Landon was improving. We just did not know to what degree, or if the improvements would stick.

Knowing he was a smart, bright kid, we wanted to see what he was capable of. We brought him in, and he was given aptitude tests by two people, one male and one female. Interestingly enough, Landon responded well to the male but not the female tester. (This may have something to do with his OCD in relation to only Ed) He fell short in understanding abstract multiple demands like, "hand me the picture of the baby next to the dad." (Landon would hand both over). In general, Landon had great receptive learning but scored weaker in the expressive language area. Receptivity, we were told, had more to do with understanding what is said to you, which was far more important. Expressivity was more language and vocabulary related. I remember the lady testing him had commented about Landon's raspy voice, expressing concern we may want to alert a doctor about that. She had no idea it was caused by round-the-clock screaming and not something we could go to the doctor to have treated. This was just not something we would bother explaining. Some things were just better left unsaid. After testing was complete, Landon was put into the IEP program within our school district, Ozona. It happened to be the "country club" of elementary schools in Pinellas County, FL that also housed PPK.

Ed took Landon to school on his first day. The Ozona rules, explained to us by Landon's teachers, were to pull up to the sidewalk and they would come and get our child out of the car. This made it easier for us and them to establish a routine for the kids, and to eliminate any kind of tear shed. They had no idea what was in store for them. I believe Landon may have been their first encounter with the type of cataclysm they were about to experience. Day one was painful all the way around. Just removing Landon from his seat was a chore. Landon's teacher, Mrs. Edwards, carried him into the school kicking and screaming that day. The days, weeks, and months to follow were worse. At pickup time we found Landon in the same condition we left him at drop off. The line of kids would come walking out of the door and there was Landon at the end of the line being carried as he kicked flailed and cried. His meltdowns at school were exhausting for both him and the teachers who had to endure this.

We hinted to the teachers to consider not giving Landon a nap. Usually after naps he wakes up in a frenzy, ready to go off the edge. At home we would always try to intercept the meltdown otherwise it's almost like having a rabid animal on your hands, foaming at the mouth and ready to bite your head off. Imagining this occurring at school without us there to diffuse it was extremely stressful. We questioned our decision to put him in school and thought maybe we should keep him home until things get better. Just driving into the school parking lot would cause anxiety for us as well as provoke Landon to cry in terror. I'm not sure if any of these teachers had ever witnessed behavior to this degree, and I'm sure those man-on-fire episodes had to be occurring at some point during the school day, especially after a nap. Mrs. Edwards would tell us we needed to try and calm Landon and try to prepare him for the ride to school. She encouragingly urged, "Make it appear fun, and maybe draw some pictures and tell him about school buses in the future." Again, this was pointless because Landon's behavior could not be reasoned with. You cannot rationalize with an autistic child. I know they were given Landon's diagnosis sheet from Dr. Kartzinel, but I started to doubt they even read it. This was a perfect example of nobody understanding that this was not behavior related, this was biochemical.

I know with Landon (and maybe with autistic children in general) there is a huge difference between tantrums and meltdowns. According to Caroline Miller, editorial director of the Child Mind Institute, "Tantrum is commonly used to describe milder outbursts, during which a child retains some measure of control over his behavior".[32] A meltdown, on the other hand, is when "a child loses control so completely that the behavior only stops when he wears himself out or the parent is able to calm him down."[33] In the beginning, when he was forcibly removed from the car, he would have meltdowns which could not be managed once set in motion. When the breakthrough happened later, Landon's meltdowns downgraded into tantrums, which were generally brought under control by Landon himself. This was described to us later by Mrs. Edwards as the greatest incident of emotion regulation and self-calming she had ever seen.

We strived to imagine a day where we could do things a normal family would, like go out to dinner, make a trip to Disney World, or Lego Land, without having to worry about a meltdown ensuing. Boy, did I really take these simple things in life for granted with my daughter, Angela. We could not experience any real enjoyment now. The blue sky, the green grass, and the singing birds did not exist anymore. If they existed, we were oblivious. I hated the world and later had to apologize to many people for hasty, emotional remarks I made during this difficult time.

During these several months after starting the new supplements from Kartzinel, Landon spent a lot of time screaming, throwing toys, and destroying the house. This made things like taking holiday photos nearly impossible to accomplish. We were stuck in the same loop reminiscent of the last 2 doctors, and ready to hurl ourselves off the observation deck. (This would be a good time to introduce a new shape to Ben. It's a circle, and it's called the circle of getting our asses kicked!) We did not know which way was up and which way was down. It was a constant process of stopping supplements, reducing the dosage and starting them back up, all while hoping to subdue his behavior. At times I thought we were getting somewhere, only to be pushed back to where we started. Landon's reactions resembled the finale in a fireworks show, rapid fire and explosive. We were so used to them, it no longer scared us. After each turbulent incident, I amused myself thinking that he may actually wake up reciting poetry one of these times.

As I sat watching television one weekend, I observed Landon walk over to the cable box and turn it off manually. Feeling stubborn, I grabbed the remote and turned it back on. Landon hollered as he ran back over to turn it off once again. I refused to lose the battle as I switched it back on. He cried and whined, ran back over and turned it off. This power play went on for what seemed like 20 minutes, until I concluded there was no winning this battle of the wills. He would have fought this war until he collapsed from sheer exhaustion.

Patterns of his irrational behavior happened so often, it came to be expected. For example, Landon would ask for an item, then scream "no!" when you gave it to him. A second later he would want it back. Yes, no, yes, no. This most always resulted in a melt-down regardless of what we did to appease him. Hope drained from my inner core each time I had to witness an incident like this. I tried to understand and had to keep reminding myself it's not his fault.

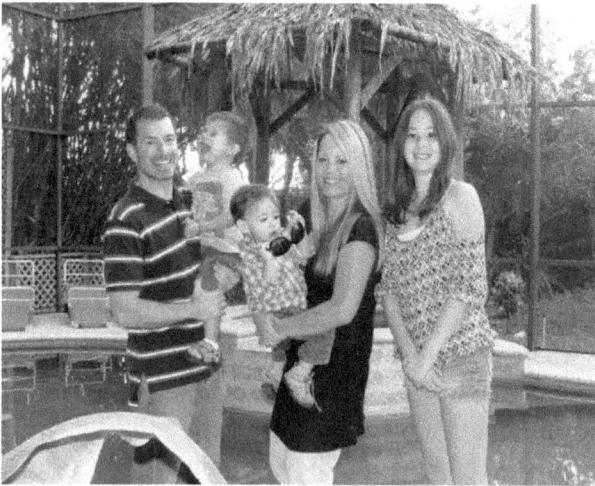

Attempted family Christmas card photo shoot

One day while preparing lunch in the kitchen and lost in my daze, I sat and watched Landon as he scribbled away on a piece of paper with that swollen, pale, sickly appearance we had grown so accustomed to seeing. I still believed I had culpability in this, despite what Dr. Kartzinel told me. My antibiotic and Prednisone use while pregnant, as well as feeding him sugar infused formulas as an infant, weighed upon my mind. I constantly reminded myself how Landon's health took a nosedive after I stopped breastfeeding. Remember Elaine from the library? She breastfed her son until age two, never giving him formula. He turned out fine. I would never live this down! Watching him was a constant reminder of what I may have done to play a role in causing this, and how we may never be able to reverse it. I broke down. Landon looked at me and asked, "Why you cry, Mom?" I was so elated to hear a question come out of him I wasn't prepared to answer. But I answered "I'm so sorry Landon. I'm so so sorry." He looked over at me, gave me a hug then said "It's ok, it was accident." Whether or not he understood why he was saying this or what these words meant was irrelevant. It meant the world to me. No words had impacted me more in my life than at this moment in time. I'm sure he had heard that sentence before when someone made an apology and maybe thought it applied, but whatever the case, it catapulted me forward. The sun poked through the clouds that day, and the tide was turning. It was just the boost I needed. I came to the understanding that if I was helpless, then so was he. One thing was for sure, he was showing more signs of development. From this day forward, I would move onward and never look back.

15

THE FINAL BREAKTHROUGH

We never gave up. Many times we thought this treatment plan had gotten the best of us and we could not possibly make it another day. Somehow during each terrifying moment, we were able to muster up strength we never knew we had. I had a little voice telling me, "not so fast, be patient...good things are coming your way". Hey, as long as there is progression, I will find a way to survive as many outbursts life could throw at us. As subtle as the improvements were, they were there. However, the regression was still present and even in the later stages; everything still seemed to go in reverse. It made us question the process. We wanted to surrender a dozen times but I would never give that advice to anyone. When we thought we could not take another step, we did it anyway, one step at a time. As things got better, it was two steps forward instead of two steps back, and gains we saw generated more motivation on our end. Then it became three steps forward, one step back. The regressions now during Kartzinel treatment, seemed less severe, but were still present. Hope was lost many times, but as they say, you have to keep on keeping on.

During these next few tumultuous weeks before our next appointment with Dr. Kartzinel, Landon spent most of the day on the iPad. He was a master at the game Subway Surfer. I was a bit confused, because from the looks of that game, it appeared you needed a great degree of hand eye coordination. This game, however, seemed to come very easy to him. He maneuvered onto moving trains, jumping up to catch coins while also moving left to right. I was unsure if this was a good sign or bad. Of course, we knew the iPad was probably not the best thing for him, but it kept him pacified through these troublesome stages.

As remarkable as this sounds, Landon decided at one point to grant Ed a one day reprieve. After the kids were in bed one night, Ed went out to relax. Hours later as I was watching television, I stood up upon hearing a sound coming from the kitchen. There was Landon standing there, awoken, all sweaty and scared. It was almost like coming face to face with a bear; in unfamiliar territory and unsure of the reaction you're going to get. Here I was, not certain of what would happen next once he realized Ed was not there. (Of course Ed was home every night, except this night.) "Come sit next to me", as I patted the couch seat cushion. To my surprise, he walked over and laid down, promptly put his head on my lap, and went back to sleep. This was an absolute breakthrough moment. It was the first time he felt assured things would be alright with Dad not there. The next morning as Ed went to pick him up, he ran to me instead, clutching my leg. He wanted Mom, not Dad! Ed's eyes were incredulous. He appeared hurt, shocked, and then instantaneously overtaken by a long overdue look of relief. From across the room, it was one look that told me the roles have now been reversed, and he will be a free man now! Without speaking, his eyes told me it was now my turn to be him. Before Landon had time to change his mind, Ed grabbed Cole and ran out the door that day...to go anywhere. As it turned out, Ed's reprieve was overturned after only one day. By the end of dinnertime, Landon realized his security blanket may escape if he did not claim it back, as he diligently reeled Ed back in. Things were again returned to normal (Landon's normal). On the other hand, this meant Landon's tolerance was showing signs of improvement, and he could now slowly start adding other people to the mix.

Landon's condition had only moderately improved, but he was still sick. What were we missing? I remembered something I had in the back of my mind that kept bothering me. I made a note to be sure to mention it to Dr. Kartzinel next phone appointment. Since we only needed one in-person office visit per year to keep him as our doctor, every other appointment within that year could be done over the phone or Skype. That day came very quickly, and what I made sure to mention changed everything.

IT'S NOT WHAT IS MISSING, IT'S WHAT IS THERE

We told Dr. Kartzinel from day one, the B12 injections seemed to help Landon but also appeared to hurt him at the same time. After each shot, some things drastically improved, but at the same time he was suffering worse in agony. Each time we stopped the injections Landon's weight would deteriorate rapidly. Only then would we re-continue the injections just so he could gain weight back. After a month of going without B12, Landon lost five pounds. He was only 30-31 pounds to start with and withered down to 26 pounds. Not only was he dropping weight, he was waking at night every one to three hours, in complete hysteria. Obviously B12 was important to his metabolic process but something about it was off. For a one to two month period, we also tried administering the B12 with folic acid orally which failed to improve anything. Landon could still not absorb B12 so we knew the injections were imperative. If we stopped the injections permanently I had no doubt Landon would not only suffer more severe neurological impairments, but also decline down to a state of immobility. Not really sure it was important at the time, I decided to why not mention the preservative.

I told Dr. Kartzinel about the time I called the compounding pharmacy and asked if there were any preservatives or fillers in the B12. I told him their response. "Yes, benzyl alcohol was used, but only a small amount which should not matter." Dr. Kartzinel immediately interjected and exclaimed a lot of autistic kids cannot tolerate benzyl alcohol and Landon is probably one of them. He immediately gave us a name of another pharmacy that makes the B12 with no preservative. Here lies the difference between an extraordinary doctor and a mediocre one. It may have been the difference between healing Landon and never seeing a recovery. I sat there in disbelief and shock. The first compounding pharmacy flat out lied to me about how they had no choice. I knew we should have investigated this further! Had we done our homework and asked another pharmacy, we could have avoided a lot of hardship and possibly saved Landon from a year's worth of torture. All those times we stopped the B12 because of his negative reactions could have been avoided. My shock turned to anger towards Dr. C for not knowing about other alternative pharmacies who offer preservative-free injections. Even after bringing the preservative to her attention, she still failed to see the potential problem it posed.

This anger rapidly diminished and grudges were soon forgotten, for drastic changes were hiding around the corner. Everything was about to turn and we were finally about to experience our first real upswing, the start of a new chapter in our lives.

The night we started the preservative-free B12 treatment, Landon slept through that night and the next two nights without incident. He was age 3 ½ now, and this is where the game changed. No supplement had markedly reshaped things for us overnight until now. Almost immediately after administering the first few preservative-free injections, a definitive switch flipped. From this point on, Landon had virtually no meltdowns, and we saw a transformation like no other occur right before our eyes. The real "happy juice" kicked in. Coincidentally, Landon's die-offs gradually became much fewer and farther between before removing the preservative. His behavior had been a lot better right before the new B12, but the tirades still existed. So it's hard to say whether the big change was due to the cleansing or healing effect ending, or if it was the change over to the preservative-free B12. This has become the biggest question I still cannot answer. Maybe it was a combination of everything coming together…the yeast battle ending, the supplements all taking effect, and the changeover of B12.

I vividly recall Landon's very last manic breakdown ending in unforgettable fashion as I opened my door one day to a Pinellas County Deputy Sheriff. "I had a complaint about a child screaming." I stood there not in the least bit surprised he was called. The only real shocker was this day had taken so long to arrive. No sooner does he finish his sentence, Landon appears right next to me with iPad in hand beaming up at the deputy with a resounding "Hi!" The deputy stares at me and then at Landon looking very confused. He had caught Landon at the tail end of his meltdown, now in a very good mood. To avoid going into unnecessary detail, I told the deputy Landon was autistic and you just have to let the rage/meltdown run its course. He immediately let out a sigh and apologized profusely, even calling me back later to tell me whoever complained never even bothered to answer the phone call back from him. There was no need for explanation. I knew it was my neighbor's son, a 35 year old ne'er-do-well, who still lived at home. He was the only one within earshot who was home at the time, and the only one most likely to do such a thing. I knew it was retribution towards me for having called the police for the numerous week-long ragers he had been throwing while his parents were away. The sound of back and belly flops off their banister could be heard throughout the night. Had I not had an autistic child who was not keeping us up all night, I probably would have joined them. If there was an autistic kid handbook, it would tell you that autistic kids do not sleep and if they do, it does not coincide with your circadian rhythm. That means Ed and I did not sleep. Having little sleep as it was with Landon up at unpredictable hours, I was in no mood to deal with parties until dawn, and eventually became driven by contempt to make the calls. Once or twice I wouldn't care, but this was happening at least one week out of every month. So this is payback? The only solace I felt after this day was the possibility of living out my smug fantasy of renting this beautiful house out to a college fraternity, if and when we ever moved. (I still have that option, by the way.) Looking back, I can put this behind me...no harm, no foul. It was just a memorable way to end that chapter of our lives. So there you have it, a police officer showing up at the door to pay tribute one last time to Landon's final "man-on-fire" episode!

With the new and improved Landon, I was now able to alternate driving him back and forth to school without a blow up. Both drop-offs and pickups became fun as he ran towards us now, greeting us with hugs and smiles in place of cries. Instead of screaming "no school! no school!", he became eager to attend. One morning while waiting for the teacher at the sidewalk, an interesting conversation broke out in the back seat of the car. Cole began making funny noises, and it was irritating Landon. "Cole, please stop", "Don't do that, Cole", and finally, "Cole, I'm leaving…sorry!", as he got out and shut the car door behind him. I laughed so hard at that moment, it brought me to tears. I laughed not only because it was a real funny verbal exchange, but more because the word "sorry" was meant as real snotty sounding sarcasm, and I was overjoyed to hear it.

This was the first time I had heard a higher level of communication from him. I loved it! I wanted more. My prayers would be answered as more was sure to come. Landon started answering questions and exchanging dialogue; a cognitive milestone in my opinion because he understood what was being asked. He also stopped referring to himself in the third person, using "I" or "I'm" instead of his own name. Sometimes he still spoke in the third person but would occasionally use pronouns when not reminded. He showed loads of affection, climbing onto the couch and snuggling up to us. He was joking around more, playing with his brother, chasing him around saying "I got you!." He began singing, something he had never done before. Every day he would go around the house singing his "ABC's," "Twinkle Twinkle," "Wheels on the Bus," and "Itsy Bitsy Spider." No longer were these advancements considered flukes to us. They were occurring more and more, and the important thing was, they were a fixture. He asked questions like, "why not?", and helped his little brother on the iPad. He was fully potty trained, accident-free. One major leap was pretend play, such as "I'm going to work, bye." All of this happening in such a short period of time gave us our second wind.

Despite the progress, we still had challenges. During this time, he still drank from a bottle, as it was still like his security blanket. Our past attempt to switch over to cups was not completely successful. We knew it remained a big challenge to eliminate this, mainly because like I mentioned before, we placed his supplements in his bottle of hemp milk. He would still not drink from a cup without being instructed to. Relative to this, we were never sure if his brain had the ability to signal whether he was hungry or thirsty, or if he would just eat what was in front of him and drink when told to. If you stuck a bottle in front of him and constantly refilled it, he would have it devoured in a matter of minutes each time.

I think I remember it taking two to three nights depriving him of his bottle before his hallucinogenic-type cravings stopped. Not only did the cravings stop but so did Landon's inordinate amount of drooling. Whether this happened from discontinuing the bottle is unknown. Perhaps it was something else behind the scenes synchronizing because a lot of things turned around at this time. Ed took it on the chin and was the brave soul to volunteer for this task. Unfortunately, Ed and I had split up at this point of the juncture, not too long before Landon's transformation. Although Landon eventually made it through, our relationship did not. We grew apart during the rough times when we probably should have grown stronger. I think we were just both so emotionally drained, seeing as that a lot of our attention went to Landon. Mostly, we just needed a break from each other and the chaos. Since Landon could now tolerate more diversity and less routine, the breakup seemed to go off without a hitch. Alternating weeks off and on with the kids would be the plan.

As the weeks wore on during this breakthrough we were having, Landon's teachers were speechless. Had an imposter disguised as an angel taken his place? One day he exited out of the car by himself before Mrs. Edwards got there, ran over to her, and jumped into her arms as he gave her a hug. The look on her face was priceless. From this day forward he wore the biggest smile, excited each morning to run to Mrs. Edwards and her assistants. They did not have a clue as to why the sudden transformation, instead they had goosebumps. How did this non-verbal, unworkable, holy terror metamorphosize into a polite, charming, warm, compassionate child who could now communicate in sentences…virtually overnight? I remember reading in Dr. Bock's book about the commonality the children he has healed all shared, each one turning into extraordinary, loving individuals. I cannot recall the reasoning behind this, but I'm guessing it's because of all the suffering they endured, shaping them early on into becoming kindhearted and sympathetic individuals towards others. I firmly believe a form of empathy and a good heart is born from their pain. This is a mini-parallel to Ed who experienced a lot of suffering at a young age when he underwent multiple invasive operations. I believe that in turn molded him into who he is today.

We always knew Landon had a good heart. Other people, especially his teachers, could never see his kindness. It was always masked by the out-of-control behavior, until now. Quickly revered as the "favorite student", he was given awards in front of the school. The principal even attended our parent-teacher conference, standing there in awe, astounded (more like dumbfounded), about the change that had taken place. Openly congratulating us, they continued to ask how this change happened, perhaps unwittingly witnessing the precise point in time that an autistic child became typical. The only regret, they said, was not videotaping how he used to behave. Even though we had many videos in the early stages to show the doctors, I was quick to remind them that when you endure those meltdowns, you just want it over with. The last thing you are thinking about is how to preserve the moment. At our low points, we also were never sure if he would recover. So why archive something that we thought would always replay itself again and again? The mere fact the principal was there at our conference told me something. She must have been involved to some degree where she had to be called to the classroom meltdowns. It makes me wonder just how out of control Landon was at school, when we were not there. No doubt in my mind Landon made the history books at Ozona, as probably the strangest occurring phenomenon to transpire in their public school system.

Even though I gave Dr. Kartzinel and Ben Fuchs most of the credit and continue to do so to this day, I know it was a team effort to make it this far. Part of writing my story is to make sure they get the praise they deserve, and to give parents the hope of healing. Ed and I laughed a lot about PPK because we were sure they always believed it was a behavioral issue, resolved by time or maybe effects of some sort of discipline kicked in. In reality, a biological miracle took place. Their eyes were unresponsive when we tried to explain the biomedical treatment process. This was just another "unpopular thing" we were talking about, which seemed to continuously be met with blank stares or complete silence. It was these puzzled looks I was given after mentioning things like yeast that convinced me it was necessary to write this book from a mother's, not a doctor's point of view. My belief is, since it is not talked about much in the mainstream, people do not give it any faith. Biomedical treatment, in my opinion, will become much more popular within the next several years, as parents start to search for their own answers. When they do start finding them, I believe it may ignite a firestorm on the medical system. Why do pediatricians not understand about yeast, the digestive system...biology? Even I get it! These questions will come up and demand to be answered. Like me, I believe when they find the answers, they will be incensed. If and when this happens, the medical community will have a lot of explaining to do. I am so fortunate to have found a doctor that did understand all of that. I could not wait to email Dr. Kartzinel after each parent teacher conference. Most of the time I'm sure he gets inundated with bad news or calls from agitated parents, but those days were over for us. One thing was for sure, Landon's immune system was strengthening parallel to his behavior. My excitement could barely be contained.

Our goal of making it to kindergarten was looking like a reality. Not only was this possible reality approaching quickly, but Landon's autism was reversing at a faster rate. Soon all the teachers, kids, family, and strangers would not notice the difference between Landon and a typical five year old. His teachers in Florida, even after being given his diagnosis, now said Landon was not autistic, he was only speech delayed. It is questionable whether they thought he never was to begin with, and maybe this was just a misbehaved non-verbal kid who had not learned to talk yet? My assumption is they did not think it possible in their minds that autism was reversible, therefore Landon had to have some other kind of disorder. The conversations concerning Landon that occurred behind the doors at Ozona would have been informative to say the least, but we would never know.

Whatever the case, we were on the right track. We wondered if this happens to all parents who have healed their children. They reverse the diagnosis in the early stages, and then friends, teachers, everyone in their immediate family, etc., all claim their child was never autistic. No credit is ever given to the parents who healed their kids, or to the biomedical doctors who take most of the abuse from the critics, skeptics, and even other medical doctors. I cannot imagine how incredibly insulting this must be, because I'm offended just listening to the cynics. Terms like "quacks" my father used to describe our first biomedical doctor was nothing more than online bait, and he took it hook, line, and sinker. It's nothing more than a slap in the face to these doctors. It's like running into a burning building to rescue children trapped inside, carrying them out on your back one by one, only to get spit on by spectators as they stand there and watch. I always think of John Mellencamp as he sings, "It's what you do and not what you say. If you're not part of the future then get out of the way." These doctors work tirelessly and thanklessly, making progressions, and pulling off miracles as they get harassed from agitators who have nothing to contribute but caustic remarks. I have a strange feeling this part of Dr. Kartzinel's profession is his goal. To have parents return back with claims from teachers and family members that their child was misdiagnosed would mean he did his job! I really do not recommend turning your back on doctors in this field. In my opinion, they are the only types of doctors who can really help you. Superheroes are rarely given credit or thanked, and at times they are even reproached for saving lives. So, keep your head up...that's just the way it is, Dr. K! The only reason for this I can think of is that our inverted society makes this possibility appear impossible. Or maybe it's because when you are at the top of your game, people just want to take you down. Speaking from experience, it's a lonely, perverse, backwards world to live in. If that comes with the territory, so be it. You may take your hits and lumps along the way but this should never deter you from your goal. This was about improving Landon's quality of life, not about trying to convince naysayers what we were doing for our child works. I would take a healthy child any day over having to be in the "right", or never getting the chance to say "I told you so".

16

TUMMY STILL HURTS

So many gains had been made, but Landon's tummy still hurt and he still exhibited signs of inflammation. I began looking into more things we could do for him. Throughout this process I felt we weren't doing enough, and explored the possibility there could be something new on the horizon to gain more ground. Supplements I read up on included food grade diatomaceous earth (DE) and bentonite clay. It crossed my mind maybe Landon had a parasite, undetected by the lab that was preventing his gut from healing. Or maybe I was just way off, and the healing takes a longer amount of time than we anticipated.

I wanted to cover all the bases so I bought the calcium bentonite clay and the DE. There are many articles and websites that discuss bentonite clay. Draxe.com has an article called, "10 Proven Bentonite Clay Benefits and Uses."[34] Made up of volcanic ash, many take it internally and externally due to its detoxing, healing, and cleansing abilities. I have heard of clay baths used by many people from all walks of life. Similar to activated charcoal, the negative charge allows it to bind to positively charged toxins. Livestrong.com has a specific article by Michelle Kerns called "Bentonite Parasite Cleanse"[35] discussing how the clay when combined with water, forms a large porous mass that sweeps the digestive tract of parasites, toxins, and even metals. It is not digested nor absorbed; it simply passes through the stool.

I tried this on myself first to see what changes occurred, and I do not recall any significant changes. Landon, on the other hand, was a different story. We had to be careful when to give this to him because it interfered with his meals and supplements. Since the bottle instructed not to take the supplement right before or right after mealtimes, there was almost no time during the day or night we were able to administer this. He took his supplements once in the morning, and once at night. His meals were given after the other supplements, which barely left enough time for this supplement to be administered. Too close to mealtime meant the nutrients would be whisked away as the clay swept the digestive tract. It almost made no sense to give this to him. I recall we tried this for a week or two before aborting it altogether. Sounding good in theory, it was not practical enough for a child struggling to maintain a healthy weight.

Next on the list was food grade Diatomaceous Earth. DrAxe.com has another article for this as well called "6 Proven Diatomaceous Earth Uses and Benefits"[36] that describes Diatomaceous Earth as a "natural product made up of fossilized remains of tiny, aquatic organisms called diatoms."[37] The only purpose I sought at the time was a parasite cleanse. An article from healthwyze.org called "Eliminating the Parasites That You Almost Certainly Have and Curing Lupus", by Thomas Corriher states "85% of Americans have parasites and should perform a cleanse every 6 months."[38] I found this article fascinating due to the fact it suggests that parasites play a role in Lupus, a widely known disease. DE is part of the list of anti-parasitic supplements in this article and suggested as "the best overall parasite treatment for humans, because it can kill blood-borne parasites as well."[39]

More importantly, the article states to only buy it in food grade form. Industrial DE is used in swimming pool filters and is chemically treated. One of my favorite go to sites is Natural-News.com for information about any health product or concern. They explain exactly how the powder works against the parasites. "DE is a naturally occurring rock made from the skeletons of fossilized diatoms, a type of hard-shelled algae. When ground into a fine powder, DE works mechanically to destroy a wide range of pests, insects, parasites, and pathogens by cutting through the exoskeleton, absorbing bodily fluids and causing them to die. Food grade DE is chemical-free and non toxic."[40]

I tried taking food grade DE for a few weeks along with Landon. This coincided with a bad decision to shock my pool with chemicals following terrible asthma from a cold. I cannot think of a more idiotic thing I have done in my adult life. After having a full-blown asthma attack from the chemicals of the pool treatment, I discovered taking food grade DE was not a good idea. The powder from the DE also may have been aggravating my lungs. Because of this, not only could I not even mix it for him, I was not sure if the airborne particles were safe. Instructions for DE were explicit not to breathe in while mixing. I decided not to use it for the time being.

After giving both of these a good try, I came to the conclusion time was the really the answer to Landon's current gut problem. I was most likely rushing things and needed to step back and let the supplements do their work. He had come so far already; there was no need to push it. The fact so much healing had already taken place was reassurance enough for me to loosen the reins and just let things be. I consoled myself with the thought that he would continue to get better as time goes on.

17

BACK TO CONNECTICUT

As school wound down for the year, Landon now age four, really started to shine. He was an absolute joy to be around, and was the best-behaved child, both at home and in the classroom. Although his diet was still restricted, and supplements were a necessity, we were not bothered by any of this. We were finally seeing the development we had waited so long to see, therefore we were willing to bide our time. Sadly, with as much care as Landon demanded, other matters had been neglected. My daughter was suffering from my lack of attention, thus not coping well in school, and her grades started spiraling downward. I encouraged her to get outside and do things, but most of her time was spent indoors on her iPhone or laptop. I learned what a brilliant artist she was, sketching better anime drawings than I have seen many professionals do. Unfortunately, colleges are going to be looking at other subjects other than art when they consider applications. Her grades were not what they used to be, and her father and I knew she was capable of so much more.

It was then my ex-husband and I decided maybe it would be better for her to finish out her high school years back in Connecticut where she grew up. She would be around her old friends and a supportive community. We did not expect the counterblast we received from her, which surprised us because all along we thought she was unhappy in Florida. She did not want to leave the friends she made in Florida. As parents we thought it was not her judgment call to make because she was not mature enough to make this kind of decision. We needed to be the ones to decide, and our decision was to bring her back to the northeast so she could finish out her high school years around her friends and hopefully shape up.

Landon's hopes for making it to kindergarten were almost complete. We had found the doctor he needed, turned his health around, and started him on a new path. In Connecticut we could still keep Dr. Kartzinel as his doctor, as long as we had one office visit per year. Ed was not happy about moving again either, as Connecticut was not a favorite place for him to live. I felt we had no choice. I still had my daughter to think about too, and this was the best decision for her in my eyes. On one hand, I felt selfish because it was a decision made based on my life and problems. On the other hand, I felt it was the only option for her.

We packed up and moved out before you could blink. Aside from meeting some nice friends, finding Dr. Kartzinel, and having Clearwater Beach nearby, I could think of nothing else positive about Florida. In the two years we had been there, we were treated like nothing more than a mark. We encountered ill-mannered, absolute "bottom of the barrel" types including multiple unlawful contractors, shady car salesmen, crooked realtors, lawyers, and a criminal dentist. In my entire life, I have never been subjected to so many opportunistic lowlifes than I had experienced in these two years in Florida. Between our last year in Connecticut and our short stay in Florida, it was during this time I had been witness to the craziest forms of illusion and deception regarding these areas. Looking back, if healing Landon came out of this despite all the deceit and corruption Florida dealt me, I would still do it all over again. I just won't be back to visit anytime soon.

I immediately made arrangements with the Connecticut school system as now I would have two kids starting in September. The teachers there were briefed about Landon's condition from Dr. Kartzinel's notes, as well as from his teachers in Ozona. He would continue on the IEP program and have a speech therapist alongside him that he would meet with on a weekly basis.. Apparently, the Florida teachers had quite a lot to say about Landon because he became sort of an unknown celebrity before even arriving. The Connecticut teachers having heard so much about him were extremely eager to meet him.

The Connecticut pre-K that Landon would attend had a mix of kids with IEPs and those without. The speech pathologist would sit with him to help with his delayed speech. I was overjoyed that this was all they were telling us he required. It was a little unsettling in a way, because if he demanded more, he would miss out on the extra help I thought he did need. I tend to overreact and think things are worse than they are, but I thought he was still far behind and needed a special teacher. Landon was about to show me just how wrong I was.

During the summer before pre-K in Connecticut, Landon was still progressing in leaps and bounds. The biggest difference I noticed is that he became not so much a "picky eater", but rather had the ability to regulate his appetite. Before, he would eat whatever you placed in front of him regardless of the amount. Now he would leave food on his plate and say "I'm not hungry", and run to the living room to play on the Xbox. He and his little brother had become quite the little wizards at computer video games like LEGO Batman and Jurassic World on the Xbox. As insignificant as this might sound to the average parent, watching what would be considered a normal everyday activity became a joy and a triumph. When do you ever hear a parent say that watching their child play video games is a gift? Watching him do anything was a gift. He was now using pronouns (out of order, but using them nonetheless), longer sentences, and had developed a real sense of humor. He became remarkably polite using "please" and "thank you" to an extreme, always doing as he was told…almost too perfect! However, being a perfect kid included never lying and that carried with it one drawback. As if compelled, he does not hesitate to rat out both his siblings when they have done wrong. Messy rooms and delinquent behavior get reported! It's very funny when it happens at home and I believe it's just his way of wanting to please us and rectify disorder. Or maybe it's just a little kid being a kid! The only concern I have is that his classmates may not react so well if this extends into the classroom. Countless people had come forward to tell us how cooperative and content he was, so little things like this is what I consider a good problem to worry about. Both Ed and I have lost count with how many strangers have approached us praising us about Landon's behavior and personality in general. I must learn to not sweat the small stuff.

School for PPK was much different in Connecticut from Florida. In Florida, he was in school six hours, five days a week whereas in CT it was two-and-a-half hours, three days a week. I found this perplexing because Connecticut is known for exemplary schools and yet only provided two-and-a-half hours of instruction. Our days were spent driving Landon to school only to go home and have to leave again to pick him up.

The first parent-teacher conference was emotional. They showed us Landon's LEGO creations and Lincoln Log cabins he built by himself. It was better than I could have done on my most creative day. The Lego structure consisted of a house, white swinging entryway fence, and a yard. This would mark the day I discovered just how talented he really was. We were told he was advanced in many areas, with only a speech delay. I asked if Landon would be able to read and write like the other kids? Puzzled, they responded, "Yes, of course". It occurred to me that day, either they were not believers about Landon's diagnosis or they never saw the doctor's notes. If they walked in our shoes, they would have understood the question as perfectly legitimate. A year earlier he was a non-verbal, unmanageable child who could not climb the stairs or walk without falling down. I was blown away! Not only did it look as if Dr. Kartzinel may fulfill his mission to get Landon to kindergarten, he may get him there earlier than expected! The conferences that followed only improved. When we met with the kindergarten staff, along with his Pre-K teachers to discuss the following year's program, we were told he may not need IEP anymore. Ed and I high-fived as we left the school that day. One more lap remaining in this race between Landon and Kindergarten.

HYPERBARIC

As much as Landon was improving, there was still one thing I had been meaning to try. While in Florida we had set up appointments for Landon to start hyperbaric oxygen treatments for his gut. Maybe this was the missing link to heal his gut completely? Landon had qualified for treatment there and we agreed to start him on a several week stint of oxygen treatments with the doctor who would perform them. It would be costly, and a little stressful, considering the chamber was small and he may not react well to an enclosed area for a long amount of time. Ultimately, the decision to move back to CT threw a monkey wrench into this plan; therefore, we could not complete the therapy in Florida. I knew there was another alternative option back in CT, a doctor who performed these treatments. However, it was someone we already had a past with, Dr. C, our first biomedical doctor.

I called her office to make an appointment for oxygen therapy. She was the only doctor in the area who performed this service. Perhaps we had not given her a chance and judged her harshly the first time. I made the appointment and felt surprisingly excited for her to see Landon and how far he had come. Well, let's just say our appointment was anything but a positive experience. We were charged a $120 consultation fee before we walked in the door. Instead of consulting with us about hyperbaric, she had us fill out a new patient questionnaire again, and rate his behaviors.

This pointless process took an hour and a half at $500/hr, without ever addressing the reason we were there. I think I might have marked one or two behaviors that still needed work on. Everything else was a positive. She went down the list and disregarded all the positive ones and focused on only the few negative ones I marked down (allergies and speech). You would have thought Landon was in some kind of unresponsive cerebral state based on the type of treatment she wanted to start ASAP. For starters, she said based on his first lab test years back, he was loaded with heavy metals. She insinuated Dr. Kartzinel's test must not be accurate (tested low), therefore we need to start him on glutathione IV chelation as well as EDTA. Without even looking at or testing current blood work, how did she come to this analysis? She told us we would have to schedule the IV treatments with the receptionist, on our way out. If we did not stay on top of this, the developmental gap between Landon and his classmates would continue to widen. Whether or not this is true remains to be seen. I can tell you for a fact Landon has only been catching up to his peers lately, not falling behind.

We were flabbergasted at her refusal to acknowledge Landon's progress. She was basing this decision on his first diagnostic lab test from three years ago. I also mentioned to her about the compounding pharmacy we used that did not use preservatives in their B12, and maybe she should alert other parents. She immediately got defensive, and blustered that if they do not have preservatives in their B12, they will soon. Needless to say, the entire appointment was a disaster. It included more supplements we had to buy from her, more blood work, chelation, and no mention of hyperbaric treatment. I had brought up hyperbaric first thing when we walked into her office. Instead of thinking over my suggestion, she talked over me and ignored the issue completely. I assumed she would eventually come around to it, but she never did. The only reason for making this appointment was to start him on oxygen, and without accomplishing anything, she turned it into a $1k office visit for chelation. I realized she did this most likely because a consultation for hyperbaric would have taken five minutes and that would not have been financially smart.

As with most stories, there is a hero and then there's the villain. I already told you who the hero is. Leaving the office, we hung our heads in shame for even coming here. As silly as this sounds, we felt guilty, as if we cheated on Dr. Kartzinel like you would cheat on a spouse and then bit in the ass by karma. All the progress he's made with us, and we had to push it. I could tell Ed was disturbed about Dr. C., and I shared his feelings. Ed is probably the only one in my life I can communicate with without having to say a word. We knew it was a mistake before, during, and after the appointment. She left us completely freaked out and questioning ourselves about Landon's positive headway. We later discussed the psychology of this woman at great lengths. She, in our opinion, is not in this business to help anyone but her pocketbook. She was only there to use her knowledge in a selfish way with parents she knows are desperate. During our visit, when she heard we had been working with Dr. Kartzinel, her whole disposition changed. That is when she mentioned the IV chelation, etc. We could not help but think she was competing with the man when they are both in the biomedical field to help autistic children.

In the end, we both wished we had just stayed away from her. She was even more defensive and argumentative than we remembered, and she did not even acknowledge what we went there for. The truth was, we were scared to death of her after this visit. She was dangerous. We left feeling we would have to go back and do the chelation and buy the supplements if we wanted to do hyperbaric treatment. Even then, I did not trust her to let us. It seemed similar to those scams where they ask you for money for the promise of a larger sum you will receive. We decided we would not double down on our investment, and instead ask for our consultation fee and our office visit fee returned. We would eat the cost of the supplements because it was a no return company policy. We later sent her a certified letter request for return of our money for failure to provide the services we asked for. We received a letter back saying "Request denied". On a positive note, win or lose, at least I will be able to give her a piece of my mind in small claims court.

18

YOU SCOOP THE POOP,
I MAKE THE SOUP

s soon as we got home from her office, we decided to forget the oxygen therapy. We needed to go back to Dr. Kartzinel for our one year visit anyway, and maybe get his opinion about hyperbaric. Ed pleaded with me not to mention how we went to see Dr. C. After considering this for a moment, I assured him Dr. Kartzinel will not care, it has nothing to do with betrayal (at the time, we really must have felt guilty, having to go to the lengths of lying to cover up something meaningless really makes the whole situation humorous now). We set up the appointment right away, and Ed flew Landon to Florida two weeks later. We arranged the trip to take place in one day, fly out in the morning and return that evening. They would call me from the office and have the appointment with me over the phone. It worked out great. What a polar opposite experience it was between Dr. Kartzinel and Dr. C.!

Landon had come so far since the last time he was there a year prior. The first thing Dr. Kartzinel said is how Landon was indistinguishable from that of a prototypical five year old. Nobody would know, not his friends, not even the parents of his classmates. At our prior appointment with Dr. Kartzinel, just one year ago, Landon was in the 17th percentile in weight, at 33 pounds. In this one year, he had jumped to the 30th percentile at 40.1 pounds. We discussed the appointment we had with Dr. C, and how she thought it was urgent we start him on chelation IV. His response to that was if Landon was in the corner rocking back and forth unresponsive then yes let's start immediately. Chelation is good if you have a kid who is at zero, not one who is a hero! We had a hero in front of us; a true superstar. He was not talking about himself; he was talking about Landon. Landon was our hero in every sense of the word.

Dr. Kartzinel's next course of action was to do more blood work. His intuition told him Landon was deficient in a certain hormone which would be detected in the blood work. Incidentally, collecting blood work was no sweat at this stage! Landon was so easy going now; we were able to do this at the lab, arm extended, with a smile on his face and happy to help out. He did not possess even a smidgen of anxiety. We would also need to collect a stool sample to test for more gut bugs. Recently, Landon had been repeating sentences under his breath after saying them and this could be a sign of a gut bug. I mentioned to the doctor this would be Ed's job. He is stronger at that than I am, and this is an area that is again a perfect example of where one partner falls short, the other picks up the slack.

When the results came back, it showed Landon's cholesterol and thyroid levels corrected themselves (all great levels), and iron levels had picked up. Since we nixed the prescription medications for those issues, I believe we rectified these levels with natural foods and repair of his gut. For his thyroid, we gave him daily packages of organic seaweed, and Celtic and Himalayan salt (natural sources of iodine). As far as good cholesterol, we mixed duck fat and coconut oil into every meal along with occasional avocados. This also indicated something very important. Landon's gut was now absorbing nutrients, meaning it was slowly healing! His blood sugar was at the bottom of normal so we would have to work on that going forward. The stool lab came back showing healthy bacteria, but it still had yeast. The amount of sugars in the kombucha is what I attributed this to, so we decided to stick solely with the kefir, regarding fermented beverages. Kombucha was really the only avenue for sugars to find their way into his body since his diet was practically sugar free. I'm not sure we will ever win the overall war with yeast but we continue our plan to fight it with kefir, probiotics, and diet. We are not sure what caused the repetition of sentences, but were hoping that it was something he would outgrow.

We made a very powerful team considering we mostly kept to ourselves about Landon. We even got the doc to agree to our assignments, Ed would collect the poop and I would make Landon's soup. On my weeks with the kids, I made Landon bone soup and always encouraged Ed to do the same. Earlier, I had mentioned revisiting this as a permanent part of Landon's diet. I now make it every week he is with me, and feed him a glass of pure broth twice a day before meals. For some reason this became my task, not something Ed wanted to add to his list. Up to this point Landon had continued with the coconut kefir, consuming approximately ½-1 cup per day without breaking out in hives. I made sure to remind Ed the allergy to coconut theory could be thrown out the window. I was now convinced beyond a reasonable doubt the hives Landon had in the past during these episodes had to be a component of the die-off. Coconut kefir is and will always be a prerequisite in my home. Additionally, I always rotate other sources of probiotics, due to the fact they offer different strains your gut needs. A few examples of what I use for us are Theralac, PB8, Saccharomyces Boulardii, and my favorite one of all...Good Belly straight shots. After using these products and having it help my intestinal issues, I thought it would be beneficial for Landon as well since he suffered from worse gut issues than I did. I cannot forget to mention Ultimate Enzymes from Youngevity, an amazing supplement Ben mentions on his show for people who have had gall bladder surgery resulting in fat absorption issues. I know for a fact I have those issues stemming from my own gall bladder surgery. I have heard him quote this product as "gall bladder in a bottle", a description straight from Youngevity founder, Dr. Joel Wallach. My intestinal issues were alleviated almost immediately after starting these, and they never gave me stomach pain like the digestive enzymes I took in the past. After learning all I have from Landon, I suspect my intestinal problems resulted from years of antibiotic use for my lung infections. Along with kefir, B12, and bone broth, these are at the top of the list for Landon now as well.

We also mentioned to the doctor that lately Landon had been sneaking bread with no allergic reaction. Music to the doctor's ears! This meant he could tolerate more foods! Dr. Kartzinel also said Landon's belly was softer now, with a lot less inflammation than a year ago. Along with the color returning to his face, this was a telltale sign his gut did an exceptional amount of healing in a year.

Physically, Landon still needed work. He was very uncoordinated, especially when running. His strides were short and flat-footed, not the same spring other kids have in their step when they run. It was undetectable to most people, but not to us. He was weak as well because his muscle formation never established like that of a typical child. This was probably why he felt like a sack of potatoes when you picked him up. He could not distribute his weight like most kids. Landon's little brother could swing like a gymnast between the table and the couch and balance himself with one arm like a ninja, however, when Landon tried this, he fell right to the floor. His strength and agility were not where they should be yet. The doctor referred to this as gross motor delay and wrote an order for physical therapy. We would share this physical therapy order with the school and they would either hopefully have a program already in place for this, or come up with the funds to start one. Physical therapy should help him tremendously for strengthening muscles and exercising areas not previously trained. These are minor things compared to what we overcame the past several years, and would work themselves out over time.

After asking questions regarding noticeable differences, one other thing I asked about was facial structure. Landon's facial structure was never quite the same after age two. At this point, I think Dr. Kartzinel thought maybe I needed a prescription for my neurosis. He hinted to me my expectations were becoming a little high, and perhaps I need to stop worrying so much over things I cannot control. I might be looking for results too quickly, and needed to give Landon time. He explained that our son went through severe neurological trauma; autism.

He gave a good analogy. When you come out of a car wreck, you will not walk the same, talk the same, or progress at a fast rate. Landon will always have some quirks. Dr. K spoke novels with the next sentence. "I can't make his eyes blue." In other words, it is what it is, and there's only so much you can do. It's not a tragedy. He was right, I really was happy, but I'm constantly plagued by the same question of, "are we doing all we can?". This feeling never leaves me; I still have it today in our new quest going forward...what Dr. Kartzinel describes as, "building a teenager."

As we ended our appointment Dr. Kartzinel said to me "I know you're going to worry anyway, but I want to plant a seed in the back of your head. He may be a little quirky, but he is going to be alright. He will be a daddy someday and he is going to grow up just fine." As he was finishing this sentence, I was beaming and at the same time ready to cry. In my head, I was already making plans involving guitar lessons, T-ball, ice skating, etc. The list goes on. I have no words to describe my feelings about things I treated carelessly and indifferently in the past. Considered by most people as normal kid activities, it was God's offering to us. This was the fun we had been waiting for, a true gift. As Ed and Landon got ready to leave the office, Dr. Kartzinel looked at Landon and said "You make me so happy." Landon walked over and simply hugged him. I believe it's moments like this where a family's most rewarding method of repayment lies. No doubt in my mind this is also how Dr. Kartzinel prefers to be repaid, not by a thank you or monetary exchange. His spirit is non-negotiable and 100% in it for this reason. It was a fantastic final lap for all of us. I glanced up at the calendar, August 15th. With the wind now at our backs, we were rounding the corner and making a break for the finish line.

19

GO CARTS, BICYCLES, AND BUMPER CARS

Our first summer back in Connecticut would be known as the first summer of fun. Landon, age five, attended his first birthday party, although he could not eat the pizza and cake. It's important we brought viable alternatives with us on these occasions so he would not feel left out, such as fruit or a piece of brown rice bread with sunflower butter and honey. Dr. Kartzinel even mentioned Landon may be able to eat pizza by next year. What fun is it if all the kids are eating pizza and he is eating broccoli and cauliflower? We were ecstatic to hear this because we had it in our minds Landon would have to be on this diet strictly for at least ten years. Under proper control, we have indulged him with little tasty treats we have added in here and there.

As far as activities go, Ed bought season passes to Lake

Compounce amusement park and spent the majority of the summer there, exploring the water park, train rides, mini roller coasters, and bumper cars. I might add, Landon's agility at maneuvering these cars is mind-blowing. He was at his happiest when he was involved in these activities. He also had magnetism about him. Little girls were drawn to him, often choosing to sit in his car right next to him regardless of the dozens of empty ones all around. As giddy as he was, sometimes he did get competitive. One boy happened to catch Landon off guard one day and struck his bumper car hard from the side. Landon did not expect this as he shook his fist at the boy and took off full throttle after him, cutting him off at every turn, and barreling at him from every possible angle. The poor boy continued to drive around remaining clueless about the wrath he had provoked or that Landon was even pursuing him. Ed dropped to his knees in hysterics wishing he could have caught any of this on video. The look of determination on Landon's face was priceless and not something we have been fortunate to see since. Our days always remain entertainment filled and we look forward to more happy rewards like these. Maybe next year we will graduate to bigger, more competitive rides. At home, he is like a professional race car driver, zooming around the yard with Cole in their green go-kart. He will throw it in reverse and back up like a driver does, looking over his shoulder as he maneuvers around. Bicycles with training wheels were also introduced this year as part of his recreation, another simple activity in life we will never take for granted again.

As far as legos go, he is a master of creation. One day on our way out the door his brother grabbed some legos to take with us to go out to lunch, something we are able to do regularly now. The legos consisted of five or six pieces that really formed noth-ing in particular. While we were waiting for our food, I watched as Landon made a bird, a boat, and a dog just by manipulating the pieces around. I was completely and utterly blown away. On another occasion after one of his friend's birthday parties, all the kids were given mini lego sets with pieces and instructions included. Watching him go to work on this was like watching a master craftsman build away. With the agility of a little engineer, he sat down on the floor with the instruction booklet open and built the entire figure formation as he leafed through each page. You would have thought he was reading, but he was really following the visual instructions. He completed the set in less than five minutes. I grabbed the box and looked at the age requirements, which said ages 6-8. The only thing Landon needed help with was opening the box and the cellophane wrapper the legos came in. Ed told me Landon had been looking at instructions and building for quite some time at his place, and even teaches his little brother how to follow them. This was not known to me because at my house he never even used instructions. I decided, why not raise the bar and really test out his skills? The following week I bought him a 747 piece Ninjago Mecha-Man creation. It came with six bags and was meant for an 8-14 year old. He completed it in two days with little to no help. The only snag he hit with this job was accidentally skipping a page of the instructions. After that confusion was cleared up, the rest was a piece of cake. It's impossible for me to come up with an answer as to how Landon went from so far behind to what I consider "gifted" mastermind levels, in such a short period of time. I go over in my head what his calling is, and I'm not sure I could pick a vocation above his capabilities. Everything now points to a future engineer!

Landon's vocabulary also continued to grow as the finish line was now within arm's reach. Cole found this convenient as he would jump on every opportunity to correct Landon's pronunciation. Annoyed, Landon would respond, "I know Cole, I'm still learning!" When he would get upset with his brother, he'd say to us, "Cole is breaking my heart." Although, not the most appropriate words for the situation, he was able to express his feelings. Several weeks into the school year I heard Landon do something for the first time; he asked a compound question. "Mom, do you want me to leave the napkin here or do you want me to throw it in the garbage?" It was the first time I had heard him communicate two opposing thoughts in his head. By the middle of the school year, he was routinely dishing out sarcastic one liners to his brother. "Cole, don't say that. You are rude!", was Landon's reaction to a name calling incident. As Cole stood outside the car door refusing to leave the playground one day and whining to no end, a little voice shouted from the back seat, "Are you serious, Cole?". I chuckle to myself at times like this because I believe Landon, mature way beyond his years, somehow skipped over adolescence and landed right into young adulthood. Every day I pray this is only the beginning. I am wonder-struck about his leaps and bounds, and he continues to advance on a weekly basis! He takes my breath away.

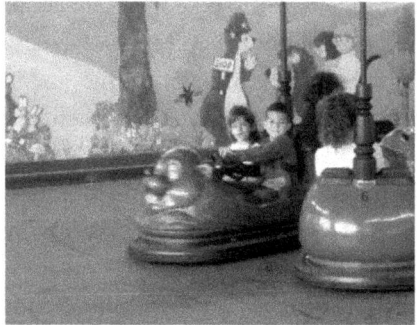

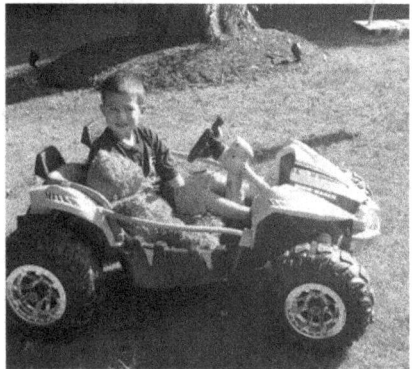

20

THE FINISH LINE

August 30, 2017 turned out to be the day we reached the finish line. Landon was five. The fact of the matter is, we had made it sooner than anticipated. Landon's broken telegraph line was repaired, and now functioning at top speed bandwidth. From the onset, even before Dr. Kartzinel mentioned getting him to kindergarten, I always felt time was a critical factor. Although we were denied the oxygen therapy, he was still ready. Shopping for school clothes and supplies, meeting the principal at an ice cream social, and going to orientation were exhilarating notions for us. We were lucky all the way around. Not only was this the perfect school environment for him, but we really hit the jackpot with having the perfect teacher. I was thrilled when I learned his teacher was Mrs. Burgess, the same amazing teacher my daughter had her for the 1st and 2nd grade.

She is the type that will give him the attention he needs, and that alleviates a lot of stress on our end.

Landon was going to be so happy here. I knew he could not wait to take the bus, something we had been talking about for a year. At orientation, he took a test run on the school bus. He walked onto the bus with all the rest of the kids at the bus stop and sat down. With a huge smile on his face, he waved goodbye. He was assigned a bus buddy to ride with him on the way home to make sure he knew which bus stop to get off at, and to make sure someone was there to greet him. Following your kid around and taking pictures every day would have become a nuisance to any child I'm sure, but not Landon. He always participated no matter what the situation was, and always with a big smile. He loved the attention. The first several months of kindergarten, I was already getting text messages, phone calls, and face-to-face compliments about Landon. The part time librarian was so impressed with how polite and helpful he was as he scurried around the library helping her clean up books and put them away. This came as no surprise to me later. I woke up one morning to find Landon had cleaned the house, putting away dishes, shoes, and toys without even mentioning it to me! Upon asking him if he did this, he just nodded with a smile. His good nature extended to a cordial demeanor when it came to conversing. As mentioned before, he was precocious when it came to manners, blowing everyone away with "please", "thank you", and "may I" before or after each sentence. If there was such a thing as overly well behaved, Landon would be the prime example of it!

November 28, 2017 was our first parent child teacher conference. Ed and I could not wait for this day, and our expectations could have gone either way. Was he way behind or right on track? Ed could sense my agitation as we waited in the hallway for a late parent teacher conference to end before our time slot. I have always had anxiety about waiting for extended periods of time and he knew that. We had a special shared alliance which could allow him to poke fun at me in these types of situations. Normally someone would tell me to relax but Ed looked at me square in the face and instead said, "You really need to take control of your candida", as we both exploded into a fit of laughter. It was funny because it was a clever interpretation that was not only accurate, but had a meaning behind it only we could understand. This little exchange set the tone for a very pleasant meeting with Mrs. Burgess. When we walked in, Landon ran over and greeted the teacher with one of his infamous hugs. He took his little brother to another part of the room to play as we had our conference. He had no modified scores on his report card. They were all C's, which stood for consistent, the best score you could get. It was equivalent to an A+ report card. The fact was, he did amazing and scored better than some classmates. She told us he is exactly where he should be, school-wise.

Landon would no longer need IEP services, except for the speech pathologist. He was retelling and sequencing stories with her, something the other kids were not even doing yet. He received a fantastic reading assessment with good one to one matching. She showed us that he was only one off from having a perfect score. In math, he was above average, now able to add numbers and count high. Like last year, he needed to work more on rhyming, although he showed signs of improvement. Mrs. Burgess told us soon he would bring a book home every night to read to us at bedtime. The children now read small words, and he was progressing right along with them.

Then she described his personality overall: "He is the best kid in the world with only goodness in his heart. He is happy, he's a good friend, and is helpful to everyone." Unanimously his classmates chose him as the child who they most wanted to play with.

We sat glowing as she described him as a "perfect child", wishing she could replicate one hundred more Landon's. She described his behavior as so helpful and mature for that of a five year old, not representative of most kids his age. She said they drew pictures for Thanksgiving about what they are thankful for, and while a lot of kids drew toys, Landon drew his Mom and Dad. We could not have asked for a better conference than the one we had that day.

Landon's speech and evaluation conference with the Planning and Placement team was not too long after the parent teacher conference, with the speech and language pathologists, special education teacher, and Mrs. Burgess all in attendance. Landon was described by all of them as "polite and respectful" and "sweetest thing in the world". As I reviewed the evaluation papers in front of me, it occurred to me that nobody knew. "I don't think anyone knows Landon was autistic.", I said to Ed beforehand, as he silently nodded his head in agreement. Landon's assessment of his core language skills was measured with subtests designed to rate his performance and factor whether or not he still needed special speech services. With some of these subtests he scored a little behind but for most he fell into the average range. His misuse of pronouns was still an area we had to work on which we met with eager willingness. The evaluation team all agreed Landon no longer needed individualized attention and would therefore be withdrawn from speech and language services. I really have to hand it to this Special Education Team. They went above and beyond what I could ever have expected out of a public school system, and were on top of everything from the day we arrived. They were just as important to Landon's milestone achievements as everyone else on our journey. I decided that the end of the meeting was the time to say something. "I'm not sure if anyone here knows that Landon was diagnosed with autism at age three." Then there was a brief period of silence. The looks on their faces told me they were never given his diagnosis papers. The diagnosis sheet had most likely been lost in the transfer from Ozona. After the moment of shock wore off, one of the speech pathologists spoke up. "You mean he was actually diagnosed from a real doctor as autistic??" For the next several minutes of that conference, we soaked up the attention this statement had drawn, as we told our story. It felt like a celebration on our part. It was a moment in time we had waited for; a time to pour our hearts onto the table and share our testimony with real willing recipients. Our conversation extended into discussions about if we were prepared to travel around spreading our message to other parents about this and we concluded that yes, we were ready to do this. This group was absolutely beside themselves, raving with us about what a fabulous success story this turned out to be. We could not believe how far he had come in such a short amount of time. We had made it, we had actually made it!

PUNCHLINE

Within this past year, my father has made dozens of compliments about Landon's transformation. He described the breathtaking change as "dramatic and undeniable". (It was as if everything said to us and how we were treated should be forgotten.) Still impressed and inquisitive about the ordeal, my father pulled Ed and I aside one evening during a holiday gathering. "So tell me what you think it was that pulled Landon out of his funk...social interaction?" This is where the audience breaks out into laughter as the punchline is delivered in humorous style at the end of a movie. Here it was, a perfect ending with satire so fitting and superbly timed, as the uphill battle and anguish of the main characters was summed up in one final statement. I guess I cannot fault him for the comment because we never told him Landon was autistic, and anyone with half a brain knows you will not bring an autistic child out of their "funk" with social interaction. In situations such as this, I do not bother. It was a total disregard for everything we've done, all the work we put in. If you think back to my comment about how I would take a healthy child any day over having to be in the "right", this is exactly that type of situation. We could explain it until we were blue in the face, and it would not matter. He either wanted proof, or his words were provocation to start an argument. I began to explain but realized I was wasting my breath as mentioned earlier. Why bother explaining this to somebody who will never know. Working in a profession his whole life with a chemistry and science-based background, I remain baffled to this day how he is unable to apply it. Failing to tie together Landon's health issues with behavior, he remains as oblivious now as he was in the beginning. I will give him the benefit of the doubt and say maybe my attempts to explain the treatment were unsatisfactory. In instances such as this, perhaps saying nothing is saying a lot more. Just agreeing with someone like this, that yes maybe it was social interaction, is the smart thing to do. (Convincing him how we accomplished what we did would entail years of re-programming the brain.) I have to give him credit though. At one point upon seeing Dr. Kartzinel's diagnostic tests, labs, plan, and what was involved, he began to see the light that maybe this doctor did know what he was doing. Truthfully admitting he did not understand the biomedical scope, he ultimately commended the doctor many times for his role in Landon's recovery. "He is doing something right." What makes this scenario more amusing than pitiful from my view, is that autism came in the door and left without him ever having a clue what it was or what happened. It's amazing to me that what he saw as a "funk" was really autism. My sister, who lives across the country in the fast and furious hustle and bustle of Los Angeles, never learned the truth about any of this until right before I started writing this book. She was painted a picture by my parents that was completely erroneous as to what was really going on. Having never figured out it was autism; they portrayed Landon as unruly and deeply troubled. With work and family keeping her very busy, she was only able to make visits every year or two. If you recall, we never left our house during these times for family holidays, gatherings or vacations, therefore we saw her only once briefly for a family photo. My brother was always a shoulder to lean on, and was also told along the way what failures we were for instituting this ridiculous, quackery-type treatment plan upon Landon, which was causing him to suffer. He never really understood what was happening with us but always listened to our problems without judgment.

The irony, and maybe the real question to be answered is, did we save Landon or did Landon save us? Had we not learned what we did when we did, our encounter with chronic degenerative diseases like cancer, MS, or ALS may have been looming just over the horizon. I was not as healthy as I had always thought, and possibly added another 20 years to my life with that detox. It was because of him I relieved my asthma, (no more bronchodilators), eradicated my lung infections, and greatly diminished my intestinal problems. I even find myself watching people and diagnosing their problems in my head. Landon helped us as much as we helped him, for we have learned to keep ourselves healthy through healing him. That is the truth. Never in a million years would I have thought autism tied into gut and metabolic problems. Today, Landon cannot be told apart from a typical five year old child. He is a regular child who likes to do regular kid activities. He no longer has OCD behaviors, his eczema is nonexistent, his allergies have diminished significantly, his sound and smell sensitivities are gone, and we exchange conversation on a normal five year old level. We remain fascinated at how he turned out the way he did. We are not entirely out of the woods yet, but I know we are close. Although his gut is still not completely healed, we continue to support the healing process through diet and supplementation. With this formula on our side, I have no doubt we will get there. Since our last Kartzinel appointment, Landon has been able to eat pizza at home and with his friends at school. Although his pizza is gluten and dairy-free, it's a huge step from where we once were. Perhaps in a year he will lose his dairy allergy...stay tuned! I am happy to say we reached our goal; we not only made it to kindergarten, we sped past it with flying colors. Landon ended his kindergarten school year with a serenade, like a happy ending to a storybook. At 5:30am my door opens and I am awoken to the sound of a banjolele. There was Landon strumming away as he asked, "Mom, do you like my music?". I loved his music. I loved everything about him, even at 5:30 in the morning!

ACKNOWLEDGEMENTS

I think a lot about what led us here. Surviving these past several years and helping Landon conquer autism was by far the hardest and most challenging commitment of our lives. I cannot speak for Ed, but in my case, this journey overshadowed any physical or mental endurance test I have ever partaken in. We know Landon's recovery is our gift, on which we intend to pay back to society. This means "paying it forward" through helping parents like ourselves who have nowhere to turn, no orchestration from their doctors, and limited resources available. We hope this book has provided you with some encouragement and information to help you on whatever journey you yourselves are taking. After going through what we battled, there is no problem out there that we feel we cannot tackle and overcome.

None of our successes would have been possible without several key people coming together at crucial moments. Let's start with Kerri on the BabyCenter forum, a complete stranger, unaware of the enormous role she played in our lives. We may not have made it to the finish line today if it was not for her. She pointed us in the right direction and like us, her conviction was strong once she learned the facts behind her son's condition. Had she not taken the time to sit down and tell her story, we would still be looking for answers. We hope she finds this book and reads it someday, like the day she picked up Dr. Bock's book. She was our guiding light and for that we are indebted. Chances are there is someone going through what we went through right now with nowhere to turn. The torch has now been passed and now it's my turn to get our message out, but from a much different platform.

I cannot forget to thank that man in the YouTube video, Michael Larsen. It was a fluke he happened to be at the office and picked up the phone that day. This was one of many things that fell into place for us syncing right time, right moment. He is an example of a stranger doing something decent for someone without asking for anything in return. All he did was offer some encouragement, but it sealed the deal for me to continue forward. This story really is amazing when you go back to the beginning and trace the lineage. BabyCenter led me to Kerri, who then led me to Dr. Bock, who led me to this man, who told us about coconut kefir, the foundation of what started our healing process. Coconut kefir was vital to Landon's healing! He was just as involved and helpful as everyone else. You know how the rest of the story branches out!

Next up is Dr. Bock, someone we are grateful towards for writing his book and then opening his doors to us. His writing served a purpose for many. My thanks to one of my favorites, Ben Fuchs for his gift of knowledge and helping us climb an incredible mountain. By now you may be asking yourself why I am putting so much credence or trust into one man's words. The answer is simple. Ben makes sense. Think of this as a book about insight and awareness. Ten out of ten times I am going to listen to someone who makes sense. He does not guess, he explains. I found that his credibility lies with his background, which is strongly linked to his ability to interpret fact from fiction in today's medical world. Overall, I share Ben's belief that you are the most important facet in helping heal yourself or your loved ones' illnesses. In our case, I believe we needed a lot of help and direction from these doctors. I am hoping there is a slight chance I am hoping there is a slight chance I changed Ben's perspective about doctors and persuaded him that maybe there are doctors out there who do heal. I can say with absolute certainty even though Ed and I played a large part in Landon's recovery, we could not have achieved this without Dr. Kartzinel's help. Ben would be surprised and perhaps happy to know that he is a doctor who understands biochemistry. Based on our experience, I have learned to tell the difference and I am now aware of ones who medicate versus ones who heal.

As you can see, in the end, we had a much larger problem than just yeast. Initially, we only went to the biomedical doctors for antifungals never expecting it to turn into something more. I may speak with a little bias because he brought our son back to us, but I consider it a blessing we ended up under the wings of Dr. Kartzinel, the found missing link in our journey to save Landon. He is a man, whose agenda was always to focus on here and now, getting Landon to kindergarten. I believe he is someone who has never been shown true appreciation for what he has done for autistic kids. Honestly, I do not think he is comfortable with this kind of praise. His son David told me his father "practices good old-fashioned medicine whether it is supplements, medication, or therapy". (Like a very own Walnut Grove's Doc Baker) But to us, he was a man of influence, holding up the house, not afraid of being attacked for practicing a somewhat controversial and non-conventional form of medicine. I compliment him on his social skills and sense of humor in particular, as he was able to bring light to our darkest moments. On occasion I was the "devil's advocate" seeking answers, yet he never got upset when I challenged him. Up until that point, most doctors we dealt with kept their information to themselves except Dr. Kartzinel, who chose to teach us as he went along. I remember Ben once talked about how the Latin origin of the word "doctor" means "to teach". This was just another characteristic that placed him miles ahead of the others. On a more personal level, he is the reason my son's eyes light up at Christmas, birthdays, and from the magic of the tooth fairy. Every phone call and bedtime story now ends with "I love you's" and hugs. This is the biggest sign for me that Landon can now live happily ever after. Whether he knew it or not, his work and his guidance was motivational for us and instrumental to how far Landon progressed. I have wondered many times whether we would have found him had I not read Jenny McCarthy's book. I believe we would have. Fate seems to work in peculiar ways, like Divine Providence. The paths may have changed but I believe the end result would have been the same. We also hope that if even one person who reads this can find some kind of reassurance or the spark of an idea to help their child, and then we will have done our job. I have been asked by some people, at what point will Landon's autism diagnosis be reversed completely? My answer is based on our kindergarten experience and is completely subjective: when you can no longer tell the difference anymore. In the end, Landon won this race. Although a bumpy ride, it was an education we continue to carry with us.

21

TO ED

The stress and challenges of having a child with autism can cause a divide in any relationship. I realize this may have been the case for us. We brought our best assets forward during these several years, and perhaps some of our worst faults. I want to dedicate this special chapter to Ed.

A firstborn is supposed to bring the happiest, most joyous times of your life. It's supposed to bring memories you want to cherish and embrace. I know it was everything but joyous for you and I'm so sorry. The experience was traumatic and heartbreaking to watch. But look what happened. Sort of like the bionic man, Landon was re-packaged, rebuilt, and handed back to us, perfect. I wouldn't trade this child for the world. You held it together at a very critical time when Landon was gravely ill and I was falling apart. An extraordinary amount of pressure was placed on you to carry us, a near impossible burden very few people in this world could have handled. You carried the weight of a thousand men. Not only did you succeed, you did it with composure. Like Landon, sometimes in life, people need to be carried. Not only did you carry Landon until he almost broke your back, you carried me as well. Incredibly, what was going through your head was never known to anyone, an asset I think makes you very valuable in his life as a father. Rarely was there ever a word muttered in complaint from you, even on those days you seemed ready to hang yourself from a tree. You were our rock with a strong inner soul, impervious on the outside.

I swore to myself I would write about this one day if Landon ever got better, and if we made it out alive. I also made a promise I would give credit where it was due and make sure you knew that the things you did were recognized. The love Landon has for you now is unbreakable and heartwarming. His head will turn at the mere mention of your name; even jumping to your defense if there is the slightest chance your feelings might get hurt. Although I feel the love he has for me, I see a special interconnection he has with you. I think you earned this bond and will find the rewards coming your way to be tenfold.

I often ask myself if I had to do any of this without you there, would I have been able to? The answer is no. Landon received the same undivided attention you gave your sick dad in the last years of his life, and it's trying times in life like this when true character reveals itself. Landon would not be where he is today if it wasn't for your patience and commitment to both of us, and for that, I feel the world should know this story. You proved that being a man is not about catching touchdown passes in the end zone, it's all about this. You are by definition what I consider to be a real man, one whose child calls his best friend. Although we worked as a team, I applaud you.

EPILOGUE

Whether you are a believer in leaky gut syndrome, yeast, B12, biomedical intervention or not, what I told you in this book worked for us. If you want scientific proof from us, you will not get it. Our evidence stands at 45" tall. Landon is our proof. You be the judge. This is just my story, a mother's story about how she helped heal her son. All I can tell you is this is what we saw, this is what we did, and this is how it worked out for us. After months of reading, learning on my own, trying supplements, treatments, foods, and finding the right doctor, we experienced a miracle. That, in a nutshell, should speak for itself. In my opinion, had we continued with the medications route, stayed with the medical doctors we saw in the beginning, and followed the path my parents subscribed to, we would not have arrived at where we are today. In my opinion, medicating Landon into a calm submissive state would not be healing him.

We saw how sick our son was. I did what any mother would do in this situation; I followed my instincts and charged forward. One thing is for sure, had I not found reinforcement from the BabyCenter mothers and from Jenny McCarthy's book about yeast die-off reactions, I never would have persisted. I can assure you they were more helpful to us than any particulars a medical journal could have provided. We were prepared for what to expect which is really what the main lesson of this book is about. Prepare yourself and read up about any information you can about your child's condition. You don't have to subscribe to the New England Journal of Medicine to find your own answers. I obtained a lot of my information from easily accessible articles online that backed up most of their facts with medical literature, while at the same time learning from Landon's doctors. A lot of these articles were even written by doctors themselves. Mostly, what they did for me was corroborate our experience, and being informed made our jobs as parents a lot easier. Holding MD licenses, Landon's pediatricians should have been able to understand the subject matter or at the very least put the pieces of the puzzle together. Ben speaks a lot about connecting the dots or adding up the clues to the story. This was a prime example of failure on the part of the pediatricians to do just that, connect the dots. It frightens me to think about how many parents may never heal their kids because they do not know of things like yeast or B12. This is where I believe the doctors need to pick up the slack and take over, not leave it up to the parents to figure out. We basically did their job for them and there is no excuse for that. What happened to us leads me to believe we have a seriously flawed medical system, and perhaps medical schools need to re-examine their field of study.

One last thought I would like to express. It disheartens me to read stories condemning parents who stood by and did nothing as their uncontrollable demonic child terrorizes a cross country flight. Please think twice the next time you rush to criticize the parent of that uncontrollable delirious child. What is happening is not always what it appears to be, and what you think is a parenting issue could possibly be something more serious. They are not enjoying the condition their child is in anymore than you are, and the child is most certainly not as well. Be smart enough to know the difference between misbehaved and biomedical problem. I was once you, and I can tell you for a fact I used to be that person cursing the parent on that airplane. To be honest, I look forward to that seven hour flight where I get the opportunity to sit that parent down and possibly change their life forever.

I apologize if this book was disorderly at times. My biggest challenge was to try and bring order out of chaos, while delivering a message at the same time. Because we're not sure of the combination of remedies that solved our crisis, we do not mean for this story to act as a guidebook or a scientific prescription for you to try and deal with yourself or your child's problems. I said in the beginning, every child is different and needs their own diagnosis and treatment plan. As I learned from Ben's show, there is no such thing as a cure for any disease. Everything is a reversal process! I wanted to write this book and tell my story mostly because we experienced so much negativity and resistance along the way. So many people were telling us we were crazy, that we believed in pseudo-science, we were failures, and it would never work. I want you to know you need to believe in yourself, in your "gut" instinct. Sometimes, it is what you see, and common sense you hear that works. As Ben would say, and I believe as well, "focus on the gut", even if it means following it.

CREDITS

Tammy K. Saunt, 'my favorite sister', Editor
Aimee Wood, Proof Reader, Editing

Ed Papapietro, Contributor, Layout
Angela Hilton, Book Cover Illustration
Christian Mayer, Photography
DougalArt, Illustrations

Ben Fuchs, 'The Bright Side" radio show
Dr. Kenneth Bock, Healing the New Childhood Epidemics
Dr. Jerry Kartzinel, Kartzinel Wellness Center

BabyCenter.com, Candida Support and Info
Jenny McCarthy, 'Louder than Words"

REFERENCES

[1] https://www.webmd.com/digestive-disorders/features/leaky-gut-syndrome#1

[2] https://www.webmd.com/digestive-disorders/features/leaky-gut-syndrome#1

[3] Kenneth Bock, Healing The New Childhood Epidemics: Autism, ADHD, Asthma and Allergies: The Groundbreaking Program for the 4-A Disorders (New York: Ballantine Books, 2008)

[4] http://hbotxofpalmbeach.com/study_pdfs/CandidaYeast.pdf

[5] http://hbotxofpalmbeach.com/study_pdfs/CandidaYeast.pdf

[6] http://hbotxofpalmbeach.com/study_pdfs/CandidaYeast.pdf

[7] http://hbotxofpalmbeach.com/study_pdfs/CandidaYeast.pdf

[8] http://hbotxofpalmbeach.com/study_pdfs/CandidaYeast.pdf

[9] http://hbotxofpalmbeach.com/study_pdfs/CandidaYeast.pdf

[10] http://hbotxofpalmbeach.com/study_pdfs/CandidaYeast.pdf

[11] Bock, p. 46

[12] Jenny McCarthy, Louder Than Words: A Mother's Journey In Healing Autism (New York: Dutton 2007)

13 https://www.jillcarnahan.com/2012/11/17/tips-for-dealing-with-herxheimer-or-die-off-reactions/

14 https://drjockers.com/the-superfood-power-of-kefir/

15 https://drjockers.com/the-superfood-power-of-kefir/

16 https://draxe.com/coconut-kefir/

17 https://bodyecology.com/articles/2-simple-steps-to-detox-mercury-and-other-heavy-metals

18 https://bodyecology.com/articles/how-cleansing-plays-role-in-autism-recovery.php

19 https://naturalnews.com/041722_coconut_kefir_health_benefits_fermented_beverages.html

20 Bock, p. 49

21 https://draxe.com/activated-charcoal-uses/

22 https://draxe.com/activated-charcoal-uses/

23 https://draxe.com/activated-charcoal-uses/

24 https://draxe.com/activated-charcoal-uses/

25 Natasha Campbell-McBride, Gut and Psychology Syndrome: Natural Treatment for Autism, Dyspraxia, A.D.D., Dyslexia, A.D.H.D, Schizophrenia (Claremont: Medinform 2010)

26 https://www.huffingtonpost.com/ornish-living/kefir-kombucha-and-sauerk_b_9750224.html

27 Bock, p. 48

28 Bock, p. 60

29 https://www.globalhealingcenter.com/natural-health/what-is-the-mthfr-genetic-defect/

30 https://www.hopkinsmedicine.org/news/publications/physician_update/physician_update_winter_2014/the_benefits_of_fecal_transplant

31 https://www.health.harvard.edu/diseases-and-conditions/the-gut-brain-connection

32 https://childmind.org/article/why-do-kids-have-tantrums-and-meltdowns/

33 https://childmind.org/article/why-do-kids-have-tantrums-and-meltdowns/

34 https://draxe.com/10-bentonite-clay-benefits-uses/

35 https://www.livestrong.com/article/320762-bentonite-parasite-cleanse/

36 https://draxe.com/diatomaceous-earth/

37 https://draxe.com/diatomaceous-earth/

38 https://healthwyze.org/reports/243-eliminating-the-parasites-that-you-almost-certainly-have-and-curing-lupus

39 https://healthwyze.org/reports/243-eliminating-the-parasites-that-you-almost-certainly-have-and-curing-lupus

40 https://www.naturalnews.com/030875_diatomaceous_earth_supplement.html

ABOUT THE AUTHOR

Laurie Hilton **is** a mother of three. Her early years revolved solely around athletics, competing in multiple sports as the only girl on the team, and earned All-American honors in '88 (soccer). She attended the University of Connecticut as a collegiate athlete ('89-94), where she competed in soccer and helped institute the women's ice hockey program. In 2000, she was named one of Connecticut's Athletes of the Century by the Hartford Courant. After graduating from the Connecticut School of Broadcasting and working a brief stint in the field of television, she and her former husband Tom, moved to Plainville, MA in 2002. It was there that Tom helped a friend start up a company called Stacy's Pita Chips, later purchased by Pepsi. After an amicable divorce sent them on extremely divergent paths, both eventually settled back in New England. Laurie is currently an Executive Producer for a motion picture thriller titled "Angel of Mine", written by acclaimed screenwriter Luke Davies. She is also a recreational poker player, competing in world poker events year round. Laurie now resides in West Simsbury, CT with her 3 children.

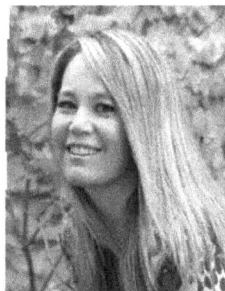

www.ingramcontent.com/pod-product-compliance
Lightning Source LLC
Chambersburg PA
CBHW060844280326
41934CB00007B/916